Obstetrics and Gynecology

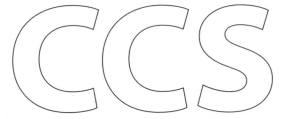

Correlations and Clinical Scenarios

Notice

Obstetrics and Gynecology

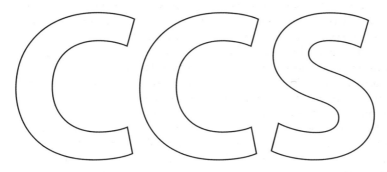

Correlations and Clinical Scenarios

Elizabeth August, MD
Chief Medical Officer of Bergen County
Riverside Medical Group
Hackensack, New Jersey

Series Editor
Conrad Fischer, MD
Residency Program Director, Department of Medicine
Brookdale University Hospital Medical Center
Brooklyn, New York

Associate Professor of Physiology, Pharmacology and Medicine
Touro College of Medicine
New York, New York

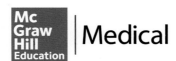 Medical

New York   Chicago   San Francisco   Athens   London   Madrid
Mexico City   Milan   New Delhi   Singapore   Sydney   Toronto

Correlations and Clinical Scenarios: Obstetrics and Gynecology

1 2 3 4 5 6 7 8 9 0   CTP/CTP   19 18 17 16 15 14

ISBN 978-0-07-181891-9
MHID 0-07-181891-X

This book was set in Arno Pro by Thomson Digital.
The editors were Catherine A. Johnson and Harriet Lebowitz.
The production supervisor was Rick Ruzycka.
Project management was provided by Shaminder Pal Singh, Thomson Digital.
The designer was Eve Siegel.
China Translation and Printing Services, Ltd. was the printer and binder.
This book is printed on acid-free paper.

Library of Congress Cataloging-in-Publication Data

August, Elizabeth V., author.
  Correlations and clinical scenarios. Obstetrics and gynecology / Elizabeth V. August.
    p. ; cm.
  Obsetrics and gynecology
  Includes bibliographical references and index.
  ISBN 978-0-07-181891-9 (paperback : alk. paper) —
  ISBN 0-07-181891-X (paperback : alk. paper)
  I. Title. II. Title: Obsetrics and gynecology.
  [DNLM: 1. Pregnancy Complications—Examination Questions. 2. Contraception—Examination Questions. 3. Genital Diseases, Female—Examination Questions. 4. Labor, Obstetric—Examination Questions. 5. Pregnancy—Examination Questions. WQ 18.2]
  RG532
  618.20076—dc23
                                                                    2014021264

McGraw-Hill Education books are available at special quantity discounts to use as premiums and sales promotions or for use in corporate training programs. To contact a representative, please visit the Contact Us pages at www.mhprofessional.com.

To my loving and supportive family: Donna August, Edward August,
Edward and Dolores Johnson, Cyndy and Joe Johnson, and Edward Johnson.
Without your unwavering support through the years, I would not have been able to
accomplish my goals. Thank you from the bottom of my heart.

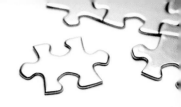

CONTENTS

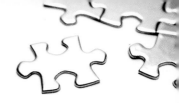

HOW TO USE THIS BOOK

The primary purpose of this book is to coach you in the precise sequence through time to manage the computerized case simulation (CCS) portion of the step 3 exam. You will find directions on moving the clock forward in time and the specific sequence in which each test or treatment should be done in managing a patient. This will cover the order in which to give treatments, order tests and how to respond to test results. All CCS-related instructions appear in RED TYPE.

If you have never seen a particular case, this book is especially for you. It never has statements about "using your judgment" because you basically do not have any in these areas. We have made a cookbook that says "Do this, do that, do this." We do not consider the term "cookbook" to be inappropriate in this case. You need to learn the basics of Ob/Gyn. Less than ten percent of physicians are in this specialty, but the other 90% need to have at least a working knowledge of it.

This book will prepare you for multiple-choice questions which comprise the majority of the exam as well as the computerized clinical case simulations and the new basic science foundations that have just been added to the exam.

USMLE Step 3 or COMLEX Part 3 is the last phase in getting your license. Most of you are in residency and have no time to study. Here is how to best use this book:

First read about the disease or subspecialty in any standard text book. We personally suggest either *Master the Boards Step 3* book (Conrad Fischer), or the *Current Medical Diagnosis and Treatment book*.

The cases in this book are meant to enhance your understanding of the subject. All initial case presentations and their continuing scenarios appear in yellow boxes. There are also hundreds of new multiple choice questions that are not in anyone's Q bank.

Every single case has related basic science foundations (which appear in blue boxes) so you will get a solid grasp of these simply by following along in the case. You do not have to consult any of your old step 1 books or basic science texts. The basic science correlates should be painless. You need not search for extra information. Just learn what we have selected in these chapters.

We always wanted to write something specifically for CCS. This is it. Because new test changes are frightening and the basic science questions are new for step 3 we made one book to cover both the simulations and the basic science.

Elizabeth August, MD
Conrad Fischer, MD

Obstetrics and Gynecology

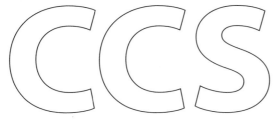

Correlations and Clinical Scenarios

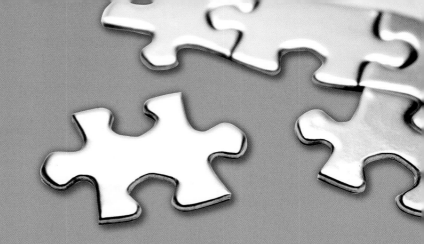

SECTION I
Obstetrics

CHAPTER 1

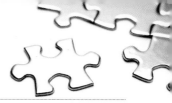

PRENATAL CARE

CASE 1: Normal Pregnancy

CC: *"I'm pregnant."*

Setting: *Outpatient office*

VS: *BP, 120/80 mm Hg; P, 87 beats/min; R, 12 breaths/min; T, 98.7°F*

HPI: *A 26-year-old G_1P_0 woman presents to the office for her initial visit. Her last menstrual period was 6 weeks ago, and she has had no prenatal care thus far. She was not sure she was pregnant until this morning when the pregnancy test result was positive. The patient denies any medical problems and surgical history and does not take any medications. Her last Pap smear result less than 1 year ago was normal.*

ROS:
- *Denies contractions*
- *Denies leakage of fluid*
- *Denies vaginal bleeding*
- *Denies fetal movement*

In ob/gyn computer-based case simulations (CCS), always do a physical examination. Even though findings are usually within normal limits, be sure to check the heart, lungs, abdomen, and extremities. A cervical examination should be done when the patient is in labor and when specifically indicated.

Which is the next best step in the management of this patient?

a. Group B streptococcus screening

b. Maternal serum alpha-fetoprotein

c. Oral glucose tolerance test

d. Pap smear

e. Ultrasonography

Answer d. Pap smear

The recommendations for Pap smear are to start at age 21 years regardless of sexual activity. However, a Pap smear is always done on the initial prenatal visit. A Pap smear as well as swabs for *Neisseria gonorrhoeae* and *Chlamydia* spp. are done together regardless of the last Pap smear result. Patients are also tested for their blood type, Rh isoimmunization status, HIV, rapid plasma reagin (RPR), rubella status, complete blood count (CBC), and hepatitis

B status. Group B streptococcus (GBS) screening is done via a vaginal swab at 35 to 37 weeks of gestation. Maternal serum alpha-fetoprotein level is done at 15 to 20 weeks. An oral glucose tolerance test (OGTT) may be done at the initial visit if the patient has a history of gestational diabetes. Ultrasonography may be ordered at the initial visit or may be done in the first trimester. However, with the patient in the office for the initial visit, a complete history and physical examination, including a Pap smear, should be done before ultrasonography.

On the CCS, the following tests are done on the initial visit: Pap smear, vaginal cultures (including Chlamydia trachomatis and N. gonorrhoeae), CBC, comprehensive metabolic panel (CMP), blood type and screen, RPR, HIV, hepatitis B, rubella, and purified protein derivative (PPD).

C. trachomatis (Figure 1-1)
- Obligate intracellular parasite
- Requires a host cell to survive
- Not visible on Gram stain

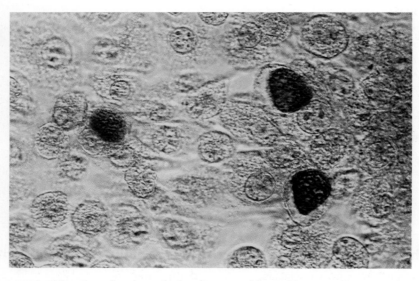

Figure 1-1. Chlamydia with inclusion bodies. (Source: Public Health Image Library, CDC/E. Arum, Dr. N. Jacobs.)

N. gonorrhoeae
- Gram-negative diploccoci (Figure 1-2)
- Grow on chocolate agar
- Nucleic acid amplification tests (NAATs) are the diagnostic test of choice

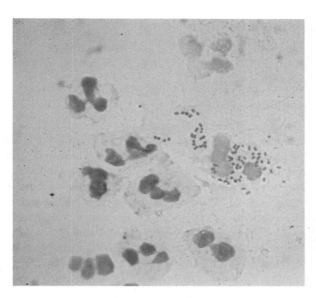

Figure 1-2. *Neisseria* gonorrhoeae showing diplococci. (Reproduced with permission from Wolff K, Johnson RA. *Fitzpatrick's Color Atlas & Synopsis of Clinical Dermatology*, 6th ed. New York: McGraw-Hill; 2009.)

> Chocolate agar has vancomycin and nystatin in it to kill off competitive organisms that may grow.

Move the clock forward to 16 weeks' gestation.

Interval History: *The patient is feeling well. She denies contractions, leakage of fluid, and vaginal bleeding. She denies fetal movement. Physical examination shows normal vital signs and an enlarged uterus halfway between the umbilicus and the pubis symphysis. Fetal Doppler tones are heard. Her initial laboratory results are reviewed:*

CBC: *White blood cells (WBC), $8 \times 10^3/\mu L$; hemoglobin (Hgb), 11g/dL; hematocrit (Hct), 33%; platelets, $250 \times 10^3/\mu L$*

Rubella: *Negative*

HIV: *Negative*

RPR: *Negative*

Blood type: *O+*

Hepatitis sAb: *Positive*

What is recommended at this time?

a. Rubella vaccination

b. Maternal alpha-fetoprotein

c. Start ferrous sulfate PO daily

d. Hepatitis B titers

e. Varicella titers

Answer b. Maternal alpha-fetoprotein

At the 15- to 18-week visit, maternal alpha-fetoprotein or the quad screen should be done. Maternal alpha-fetoprotein is a part of the quad screen, which also includes beta-human chorionic gonadotropin (β-HCG), estriol, and inhibin A. The results of all four tests are needed to interpret if the patient has an increased risk of Down syndrome. Abnormalities are associated with complications in pregnancy, such as Down syndrome, neural tube defects, and abnormal anatomy. However, the most common reason for an abnormality is a dating error. If an abnormality is detected, either elevated or decreased, ultrasonography should be done. Multiple gestations and anatomical abnormalities (e.g., neural tube defects) increase the maternal alpha-fetoprotein level. Down syndrome is associated with a low alpha-fetoprotein level (Figure 1-3).

Rubella vaccination is not done during pregnancy. All live vaccines are *contraindicated* during pregnancy. The flu shot and Tdap (diphtheria, tetanus, and pertussis) are recommended during pregnancy. They are safe pregnant patients' children may receive live vaccinations, such as varicella or MMR (measles, mumps, and rubella). Viral shedding does occur, but the children cannot transmit the virus to their pregnant mothers. Hepatitis titers are not needed in this mother. She is hepatitis B surface antibody positive. This is consistent with being immune to hepatitis. Varicella titers are not needed because the vaccine cannot be given to a pregnant woman.

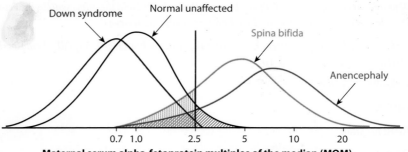

Alpha-fetoprotein
• Produced by yolk sac
• Liver of fetus

Figure 1-3. Maternal alpha-fetoprotein and the most common abnormalities seen. (Reproduced with permission from Cunningham F, Leveno K, Bloom S, et al. *Williams Obstetrics*, 23rd ed. New York: McGraw-Hill; 2010.)

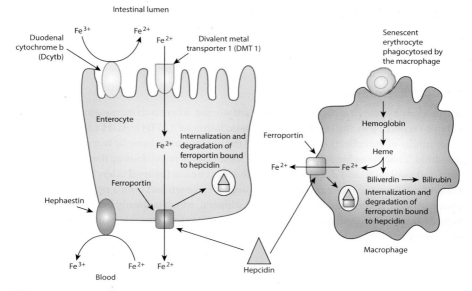

Figure 1-4. Biochemistry of how hepcidin inhibits transportation of iron. Pregnant women require more iron than hepcidin allows transport of. (Reproduced with permission from Murray RK, Bender DA, Botham KM, Kennelly PJ, Rodwell VW, Weil PA. *Harper's Illustrated Biochemistry*, 29th ed. New York: McGraw-Hill; 2012.)

ADH ↑

↑ Hepcidin

Why are all pregnant women iron deficient?

a. Decreased absorption
b. Decreased intake

c. Increased hepcidin
d. Decreased ferric reductase

Answer c. Increased hepcidin

Hepcidin is a protein that is produced by the liver that inhibits transportation of iron (Figure 1-4). It only allows absorption of about 4 to 5 mg per day. Pregnant women have an increase demand for iron, and hepcidin prevents its absorption.

Where is iron absorbed?

a. Stomach
b. Duodenum

c. Jejunum
d. Ileum

Answer b. Duodenum

The duodenum absorbs the cations from the diet, such as iron (Fe^{++}), calcium (Ca^{++}), and magnesium (Mg^{++}). This is why patients with celiac disease are iron deficient. They have no microvilli.

What is the mechanism of anemia in pregnancy?

a. Iron malabsorption
b. Folate malabsorption
c. Increased ADH

d. Excess aldosterone
e. Decreased permeability of the collecting duct

Answer c. Increased ADH

Anemia is a physiological change in all pregnant women. There is an increase in blood plasma volume secondary to the increased antidiuretic hormone (ADH). ADH causes increased permeability of the collecting duct and resets the hypothalamic osmolar receptor to a higher threshold. This allows for the patient's blood volume to increase, diluting the red blood cells. This is physiological and does not require treatment unless the level is less than 10 mg/dL. Prenatal vitamins are recommended in all pregnant women and have a significant amount of iron. Adding ferrous sulfate may cause constipation, which is already a common problem in pregnancy. Pregnant women are anemic secondary to the increase in plasma volume from an increase in ADH and are iron deficient secondary to the increase in hepcidin.

Move the clock forward 1 week.

Interval History: *The patient calls the office concerned about the hepatitis antibody.*

What does hepatitis surface antibody positive signify?

a. She is immune, and no further action is required.
b. Repeat the test in 6 to 8 weeks.

c. Advise her to have infant IVIG at birth.
d. Administer hepatitis B vaccine.

Answer a. She is immune, and no further action is required.

Surface antibodies mean that the patient is immune to hepatitis B; no further action is needed for the mother or the infant.

What type of antibody is hepatitis B surface antibody?

a. IgM
b. IgG

c. IgA
d. IgE

Answer b. IgG (Figure 1-5)

Hepatitis B surface antibody is an IgG that can pass through the placenta and provide some immunity to the baby. Similar to all IgG antibodies that pass to the infant, it will last for about 6 months.

Move the clock forward to 25 weeks' gestation.

Interval History: *The patient is feeling well and denies contractions, leakage of fluid, and vaginal bleeding. She states that she feels the baby moving often. Her prenatal care is up to date, and there are no complications.*

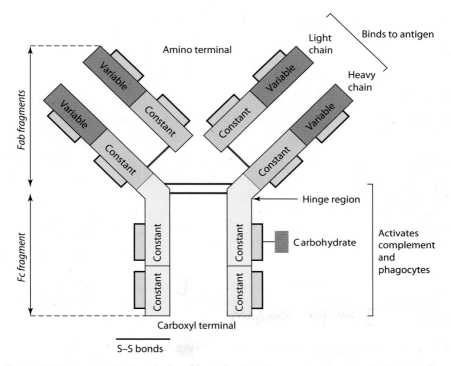

Figure 1-5. Structure of IgG antibodies. (Reproduced with permission from Brooks GF, Carroll KC, Butel J, Morse S. *Jawetz, Melnick, & Adelberg's Medical Microbiology*, 26th ed. New York: McGraw-Hill; 2013.)

What the next step in the management of this patient?

a. Administration of RhoGAM
b. Group B streptococcus screening
c. *N. gonorrhoeae* screening

d. 1-hour glucose tolerance test
e. Maternal alpha-fetoprotein level

Answer d. 1-hour glucose tolerance test

Gestational diabetes is a common prenatal complication. Gestational diabetes is screened for in all asymptomatic pregnant women between 24 and 28 weeks of gestation. The pregnant woman drinks 50 g of glucose and has her blood sugar level checked 1 hour later. If this level is more than 130 mg/dL, the patient should be sent for the 3-hour OGTT. The 1-hour OGTT is a screening test that is done regardless of the patient's last meal. It is not necessary to fast for the 1-hour OGTT.

If the 1-hour OGTT yields an abnormal result, a 3-hour OGTT should be done (Figure 1-6). The patient is required to fast overnight and drink 100 g of glucose. The patient will then undergo several blood glucose levels: fasting (>95 mg/dL), 1 hour (>180 mg/dL), 2 hours (>155 mg/dL), and 3 hours (>140 mg/dL). If two of the blood sugar levels are more than the indicated levels, then gestational diabetes is diagnosed.

RhoGAM would be administered at 28 weeks of gestation if the mother was Rh negative. The question would clue you into this diagnosis if the answer is RhoGAM. For

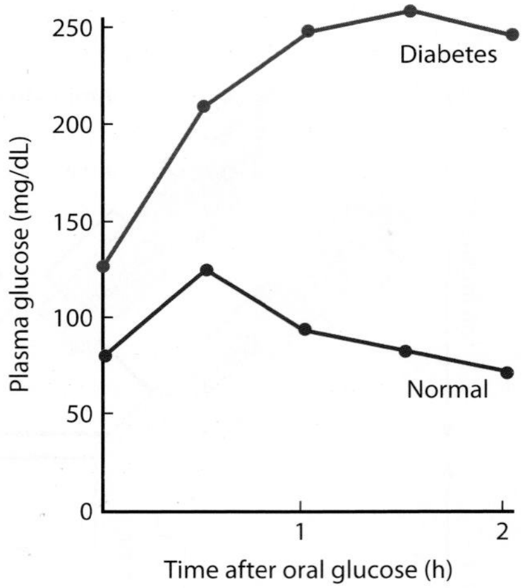

Figure 1-6. Glucose tolerance test results on normal patients versus patients with diabetes. (Reproduced with permission from Barrett KE, Barman SM, Boitano S, Brooks H. *Ganong's Review of Medical Physiology,* 24th ed. New York: McGraw-Hill; 2012.)

example, the question would include that the patient had to have an injection after an episode of vaginal bleeding, that she was Rh negative or that she previously had a baby with hydrops fetalis.] Clue for RhoGAM

GBS screening is done at 36 weeks of gestation. If the patient had GBS during this pregnancy at any point (in urine, vaginal secretions during the first trimester, or on screen at 36 weeks), she will need antibiotic treatment during labor. If the patient had a baby who was affected by GBS, the patient should be treated during labor. GBS can cause sepsis in newborns.

Screening for *N. gonorrhoeae* is done at the initial visit.

Maternal alpha-fetoprotein levels are done between 16 and 18 weeks of gestation.

Screening test vs. specific test

Screening test = very sensitive
• It needs to be able to detect all patients that may have the disease.
• Sensitivity = true positives/true positives + false negatives

Confirmatory tests = very specific
• Detect all people who actually have the disease
• Specificity = true negatives/true negatives + false positives

What causes gestational diabetes?

a. Obesity or weight gain
b. Pancreatic insulin deficiency

c. Human placental lactogen (HPL)
d. Prolactin blocks insulin

Answer c. Human placental lactogen (HPL)

HPL is an anti-insulin for the mother. It tips genetically predisposed women into diabetes during pregnancy. HPL is a hormone that has no function under normal gestational conditions. Under conditions of starvation, it preserves food for the fetus. As an anti-insulin for the mother, it blocks glucose and free fatty acids being picked up by the maternal cells so that the fetus will pick up the glucose and free fatty acids.

Move the clock forward to 36 weeks' gestation.

Interval History: *The patient is feeling well and denies contractions, leakage of fluid, and vaginal bleeding. The patient states that the baby is moving constantly. Vital signs show a blood pressure of 130/80 mm Hg, heart rate of 85 beats/min, and respiratory rate of 14 breaths/min. Physical examination is significant for a fundal height of 35 cm and fetal heart rate in the 160s.*

Which is next best step in the management of this patient?

a. Send to L&D for evaluation of preeclampsia

b. 24-hour urine

c. Vaginal culture for group B streptococcus (GBS)

d. Ultrasonography

Answer c. Vaginal culture for group B streptococcus (GBS).

GBS (Figure 1-7) sepsis in a neonate is a feared complication among women who are asymptomatic carriers of the bacteria. Sepsis is preventable if the woman is given antibiotics during labor. All women should have a vaginal and rectal swab for GBS at 36 weeks of gestation.

What is GBS?

a. A gram-positive cocci

b. An enterococci

c. A gram-negative diplococci

d. A gram-negative coccobacilli

e. *Viridans* group streptococci

Answer a. A gram-positive cocci.

Examples of gram-positive rods are *Clostridium* and *Bacillus* spp. A gram-negative diplococci is *N. gonorrhoeae* (see Figure 1-2). Examples of gram-negative rod include *Klebsiella* spp., *Escherichia coli*, and *Pseudomonas* spp. Gram-negative coccobacilli (Figure 1-8) include *Haemophilus influenzae*, *Bordetella pertussis*, and *Brucella* spp. Although enterococci and *Viridans* group streptococci are gram-positive cocci, they do not cause perinatal complications. The other name for it is *Streptococcus agalactiae*.

Streptococcal bacteria are classified into Lance-field groups based on the polysaccharide antigens on the cell wall.

Vaginal and rectal GBS screening cultures at 35–37 weeks' gestation for ALL pregnant women (unless patient had GBS bacteriuria during the current pregnancy or a previous infant with invasive GBS disease)

Intrapartum prophylaxis indicated

- Previous infant with invasive GBS disease

- GBS bacteriuria during current pregnancy

- Positive GBS screening culture during current pregnancy (unless a planned cesarean delivery, in the absence of labor or amniotic membrane rupture, is performed)

- Unknown GBS status (culture not done, incomplete, or results unknown) and any of the following:

  - Delivery at <37 weeks' gestation

  - Amnionic membrane rupture ≥18 hours

  - Intrapartum temperature ≥100.4°F (≥38.0°C)

Intrapartum prophylaxis not indicated

- Previous pregnancy with a positive GBS screening culture (unless a culture was also positive during the current pregnancy)

- Planned cesarean delivery performed in the absence of labor or membrane rupture (regardless of maternal GBS culture status)

- Negative vaginal and rectal GBS screening culture in late gestation during the current pregnancy, regardless of intrapartum risk factors

Figure 1-7. Indications for intrapartum treatment of group B streptococcus (GBS). (Reproduced with permission from Cunningham F, Leveno K, Bloom S, et al. *Williams Obstetrics,* 23rd ed. New York: McGraw-Hill; 2010; Adapted from Centers for Disease Control and Prevention, 2002.)

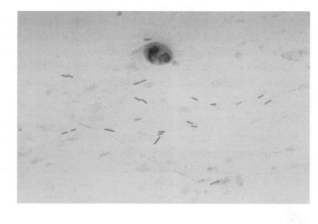

Figure 1-8. Gram-negative coccobacilli. (Reproduced with permission from Knoop KJ, Stack L, Storrow A, Thurman RJ. *The Atlas of Emergency Medicine,* 3rd ed. New York: McGraw-Hill; 2010.)

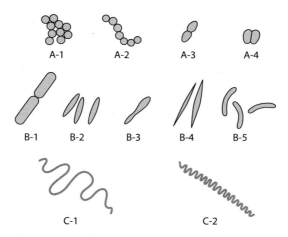

Figure 1-9. Bacterial morphology. A are cocci, and B are bacilli. (Modified and reproduced with permission from Joklik WK. *Zinsser Microbiology,* 20th ed. Originally published by Appleton & Lange. Copyright 1992 by McGraw-Hill.)

- Gram positive = purple (retains the stain) (Figure 1-9)
- Gram negative = red (does not retain stain)

- Cocci = circular shape
- Bacilli = rod shape

Move the clock forward 1 week.

Interval History: *The patient presents to labor and delivery for leakage of fluid at 38 weeks' gestation. She has been having lower abdominal pain for 2 hours that is intermittent and severe. She suddenly felt a gush of fluid from her vagina. The baby has been moving. Results of the vaginal culture were positive.*

Which of the following is the next step in the management of this patient?

a. Administer amoxicillin IV

b. Manual examination of the cervix

c. Nitrazine test

d. Fetal fibronectin

Answer c. Nitrazine test

Amniotic fluid is alkaline. Vaginal fluid is acidic. If nitrazine indicates the fluid has a pH of 7, then it is likely amniotic fluid. When amniotic fluid dries, it also causes a ferning pattern on a slide, so that may also be indicated. Normal vaginal pH is 4.5.

Amoxicillin will need to be administered if the patient is truly in labor. However, the fluid must first be confirmed as amniotic fluid.

Manual examination of the cervix will need to be done, but a sterile speculum examination should be done first to assess the fluid. One would like to observe the fluid to see if it is collected in the posterior fornix. The fluid would also need to be sampled for testing with nitrazine paper.

Fetal fibronectin leaks into the vagina. Test for fibronectin when preterm labor is being considered. A negative test result for fibronectin makes preterm labor unlikely.

Nitrazine paper
• Determines pH
• Changes color based on pH
• Detects a pH of 4.5 to 7.5

Nitrazine paper is positive for amniotic fluid. The patient is in labor. "Positive" means a pH > 6.0

CASE 2: Advanced Maternal Age

CC: *"I'm 38 years old and pregnant."*

Setting: *Outpatient clinic*

VS: *BP, 123/75 mm Hg; P, 75 beats/min; R, 13 breaths/min; T, 98.4°F*

HPI: *A 38-year-old woman with an intrauterine pregnancy at 16 weeks' gestation presents to the office for a routine prenatal visit. The patient states that she had her maternal alpha-fetoprotein level checked last week. She states that the resident told her that the level was elevated. She would like further evaluation.*

Which of the following is the next step in the management of this patient?

a. Amniocentesis

b. Chorionic villus sampling

c. Cordocentesis

d. Repeat maternal alpha-fetoprotein

e. Ultrasonography

Answer e. Ultrasonography

The most common reason for an abnormality in the maternal alpha-fetoprotein is a dating error. Ultrasonography is always done to confirm the dates of gestation and to monitor for anatomical abnormalities. However, the woman may opt to have an amniocentesis because she has an advanced maternal age.

Amniocentesis is done in the second trimester between 16 and 20 weeks' gestation (Figure 1-10). A needle is inserted through the abdomen into the amniotic sac. Amniotic fluid is aspirated and sent for karyotyping. Amniocentesis holds many risks such as direct fetal injury, indirect fetal injury, leakage of amniotic fluid, rupture of membranes, and fetal loss. Women age 35 years and older are considered as having advanced maternal age. These women should be offered amniocentesis or chorionic villus sampling (CVS) in the first trimester to detect any genetic abnormalities.

CVS is a procedure that is done in the first trimester (Figure 1-11). It takes transvaginal samples of the chorionic villi and sends them for karyotyping. This approach is done after 10 weeks' gestation. Patients are at increased risk for both direct fetal injury and fetal loss.

Cordocentesis or percutaneous cord blood sampling is done if the fetus needs a blood transfusion or her acid–base status needs to be determined (Figure 1-12). This is a very risky procedure and carries a high risk of fetal loss.

Repeating maternal alpha-fetoprotein testing is possible after confirming the dates, anatomy, and gestation by ultrasonography.

Chorionic villi are a part of the placenta. They are the border between maternal and fetal circulation.

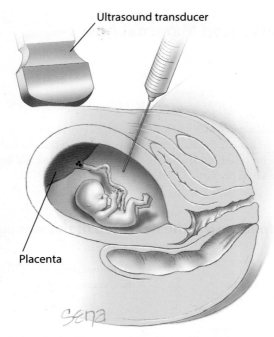

Figure 1-10. Amniocentesis. (Reproduced with permission from Cunningham F, Leveno K, Bloom S, et al. *Williams Obstetrics*, 23rd ed. New York: McGraw-Hill; 2010.)

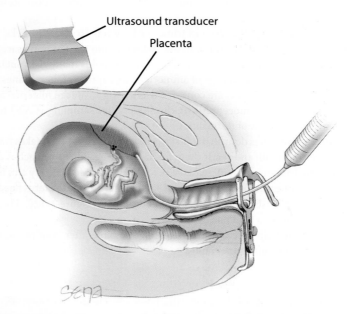

Figure 1-11. Chorionic villus sampling. (Reproduced with permission from Cunningham F, Leveno K, Bloom S, et al. *Williams Obstetrics*, 23rd ed. New York: McGraw-Hill; 2010.)

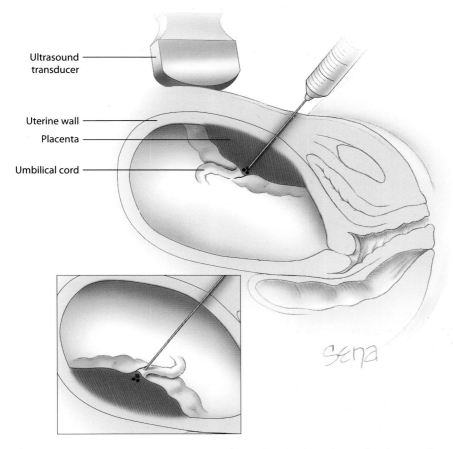

Ultrasound transducer

Uterine wall

Placenta

Umbilical cord

Figure 1-12. Percutaneous fetal blood sample. (Reproduced with permission from Cunningham F, Leveno K, Bloom S, et al. *Williams Obstetrics,* 23rd ed. New York: McGraw-Hill; 2010.)

Interval History: *Ultrasonography revealed that there was a dating error and the fetus was smaller than previously thought. No anatomical abnormalities were noted. If abnormities were noted on the ultrasonography, more invasive testing such as amniocentesis or CVS may be done.*

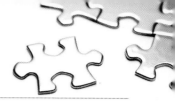

CHAPTER 2

MATERNAL DISEASE DURING PREGNANCY

CASE 1: Maternal Hypertension

CC: *"I'm pregnant."*

Setting: *Outpatient office*

VS: *BP, 155/90 mm Hg; P, 85 beats/min; R, 12 breaths/min; T, 98°F*

HPI: *The patient is a 25-year-old G_1P_0 with an intrauterine pregnancy (IUP) at 24 weeks' gestation. She presents for her routine prenatal checkup. She has never had problems with blood pressure (BP). At her previous visit, her BP was 160/90 mm Hg.*

ROS:
- *Denies chest pain*
- *Denies shortness of breath*
- *Denies headache and blurry vision*
- *Denies abdominal pain and contractions*
- *Denies leakage of fluid*
- *Denies vaginal bleeding*
- *Fetal movement: present*

Physical Exam:
- *Cardiovascular: S_1S_2+ RRR no m/r/g*
- *Lung: CTA bilaterally*
- *Extremities: 1+ edema*
- *Fundal height: 23 cm*
- *Fetal heart rate: 150s*

What is the next step in the management of this patient?

a. Start lisinopril.

b. Perform renal ultrasonography.

c. Check urine dipstick.

d. Observe BP.

e. Prescribe hydrochlorothiazide.

Answer c. Check urine dipstick.

Proteinuria may be a sign of preeclampsia, eclampsia, or a hydatiform mole. All pregnant patients who have an elevated BP should have a urine dipstick done first. Because there are no symptoms, it is not urgent to start antihypertensive medications immediately. If there were proteinuria, treatment becomes more urgent. There is nothing on a renal ultrasound that will tell you this is eclampsia.

On the CCS, the initial order set for this patient should include:

- BP
- Urine dipstick
- Comprehensive metabolic panel (CMP)

Move clock forward to the next laboratory test result.

Urine dipstick was done and shows no proteinuria. BP continues to be elevated at 150/90 mm Hg.

What is the next step in the management of this patient?

a. Start lisinopril.
b. Start labetalol.
c. Continue to observe BP.

d. Send to the labor and delivery department.
e. Conduct ultrasonography.

Answer b. Start labetalol.

Labetalol has both α- and β-adrenergic blocking activity. This may allow for greater utero-placental blood flow compared with β-blockers alone. Lisinopril is contraindicated in pregnancy. Treatment with antihypertensive drugs is needed if BP is consistently above 150/90 mm Hg in pregnancy. Delivery of a 24-week fetus is nearly universally fatal to the infant. Survival begins around 25 or 26 weeks. In addition, the absence of proteinuria means this is not eclampsia.

Classification of hypertension:
- Chronic: Starts *before* 20 weeks' gestation
- Gestational: Starts *after* 20 weeks' gestation
- Preeclampsia with proteinuria
- Eclampsia with proteinuria *and seizures*
- HELLP syndrome: Hemolysis, elevated liver enzymes, low platelets

---

Which of the following drugs is contraindicated in gestational hypertension?

a. Methyldopa
b. Nifedipine

c. Nitroprusside
d. Hydralazine

Answer c. Nitroprusside

Nitroprusside is contraindicated in pregnant patients because of possible fetal cyanide poisoning. Calcium channel blockers such as nifedipine are safe in pregnancy.

Pharmacology drug classes:
- Class A: Good in pregnancy; good studies show no risk
- Class B: Acceptable in pregnancy, animal studies show no risk, but no human studies have been conducted. Most drugs considered "SAFE" in pregnancy are class B, not class A.
- Class C: If the benefits outweigh the risk, then acceptable in pregnancy. Animal studies show adverse effects; no human studies have been conducted.
- Class D: Adverse effects in human studies
- Class X: Contraindicated in pregnancy: Definitely teratogenic

Three days after starting labetalol, the patient returns to the office for a BP check. Her BP is now 132/84 mm Hg. Continue to see the patient at 2- to 4-week intervals to assess her BP during pregnancy. You will not know until after the delivery whether the hypertension will resolve.

CASE 2: Diabetes in Pregnancy

CC: *"I'm pregnant and have diabetes."*

Setting: *Outpatient office*

VS: *BP, 120/80 mm Hg; P, 75 beats/min; R, 12 breaths/min; T, 98°F*

HPI: *A 32-year-old woman with a history of diabetes presents with an IUP at 5 weeks. She has been taking metformin, glyburide, and lisinopril. Her glucose has been well controlled on these medications.*

ROS:
- *Denies leakage of fluid*
- *Denies contractions*
- *Denies fetal movement*
- *Denies vaginal bleeding*
- *Denies abdominal pain*

What is the next best step in the management?

a. Switch the patient to insulin.
b. Continue metformin but discontinue glyburide.
c. Continue both metformin and glyburide.
d. Stop both metformin and glyburide and change to acarbose.
e. Stop both metformin and glyburide and start rosiglitazone.

Answer a. Switch the patient to insulin.

In all pregnant patients, the treatment of choice is insulin. If the patient adamantly refuses insulin, then glyburide can be continued. Metformin is discontinued in the first trimester but may be given in the second and third trimesters. However, if the patient is taking metformin for polycystic ovary syndrome (PCOS), metformin should be continued during the first trimester. In PCOS, metformin restores fertility by an unknown mechanism. Metformin and glyburide are the only acceptable oral therapies at this time, and even they should only be used if insulin cannot be given. Acarbose and rosiglitazone are not recommended at this time.

On the CCS, the initial order set should include discontinuation of the angiotensin-converting enzyme (ACE) inhibitor and metformin, HgbA1c, and CMP.

Incretins are:
- Glucagon-like peptide (GLP)
- Glucose insulinotropic peptide (GIP)
- Increase insulin release from pancreas

Which class does metformin belong to?

a. Sulfonylurea

b. Thiazolidinediones

c. Meglitinides

d. α-Glucosidase inhibitors

e. Biguanide

Answer e. Biguanide

A biguanide works via decreasing hepatic glucose production and decreasing intestinal absorption. Metformin blocks gluconeogenesis. They do not cause hypoglycemia. α-Glucosidase inhibitors such as acarbose work by blocking the intestinal absorption of glucose.

What is the mechanism of action of glyburide?

a. Increase in insulin sensitivity

b. Activate the nuclear peroxisome proliferator-activated receptor gamma (PPAR-γ)

c. Secretagogue

d. GLP-1 analog

e. Dipeptidyl peptidase 4 (DPP-4) inhibitor

Answer c. Secretogogues

Glyburide is a sulfonylurea. Sulfonylureas block the potassium channel in the pancreatic β cells. This causes a change in the resting potential of the cell via an influx of calcium ions and causes the cell to secrete insulin. Biguanides increase insulin sensitivity. Thiazolidinediones activate the nuclear PPAR-γ. GLP-1 analogs are a class of drugs that include exenetide and liraglutide. DPP-4 inhibitors are a class of drugs that include sitagliptin, saxagliptin, and linagliptin. Rosiglitazone and pioglitazone are activators of the nuclear PPAR. They increase peripheral insulin sensitivity.

Sulfonylureas block potassium egress (leaving) β cells.
Increased potassium in β cells depolarizes β cells.
Depolarized β cells release insulin.

DPP-4 inhibitors:
• Block metabolism of "incretins"
• Incretins increase insulin release and decrease glucagon

What is the definition of gestational diabetes?

a. Type I diabetes

b. Type II diabetes before pregnancy

c. Glucose intolerance *before* 20 weeks' gestation that does not resolve

d. Glucose intolerance *before* 20 weeks' gestation that resolves by 6 weeks postpartum

e. Glucose intolerance *after* 20 weeks' gestation that resolves by 6 weeks postpartum

f. Type I diabetes *after* 20 weeks' gestation that does not resolve

Answer e. Glucose intolerance *after* 20 weeks' gestation that resolves by 6 weeks postpartum

Gestational diabetes is defined as glucose intolerance that starts after 20 weeks' gestation and resolves by 6 weeks' postpartum. It is diagnosed with a fasting glucose of greater than or equal to 92 mg/dL but less than or equal to 126 mg/dL. It may also be diagnosed on the oral glucose tolerance test at 24 to 28 weeks' gestation.

Overt diabetes is diabetes type I or II that occurred before the patient became pregnant. Overt diabetes can be diagnosed with:

• HgbA1c greater than or equal to 6.5 mg/dL
• Fasting glucose more than 126 mg/dL on two occasions
• Symptomatic with random glucose level greater than 200 mg/dL

Mothers with gestational diabetes are at increased risk for developing type II diabetes later in life.

Move the clock forward 4 weeks.

Setting: *Outpatient office*

Interval History: *The patient has received normal prenatal care. She monitors her glucose levels and has been strictly maintained with insulin. Her pregnancy is at 32 weeks of gestation. She denies vaginal bleeding, leakage of fluid, and contractions. The baby is moving well.*

What is the next step in the management of this patient?

a. Weekly ultrasonography
b. Ultrasonography twice a week
c. Weekly biophysical profile (BPP)
d. Weekly nonstress test
e. Nonstress test twice a week

Answer e. Nonstress test twice a week

There is an increase in mortality rates in children of mothers with diabetes. They need to be monitored closely for decelerations in their heart rate. This should be done with twice-weekly nonstress tests or BPPs. Ultrasonography may be done to monitor growth but not on a weekly or twice-weekly basis. A BPP is ultrasonography and a nonstress test done together to assess the fetus' well-being and growth. It measures fetal movement, fetal tone, fetal breathing, and amniotic fluid index, and includes a nonstress test.

What is the main concern for the fetus at this time?

a. Neonatal hypoglycemia
b. Hyperbilirubinemia
c. Macrosomia
d. Hypercalcemia

Answer c. Macrosomia

During pregnancy, the main concern is if the fetus is getting too big. Many complications of pregnancy are related to fetal size and weight. Premature infants weight too little. Infants of mothers with diabetes are too large (Figure 2-1). Hypoglycemia, hyperbilirubinemia, hypercalcemia are all complications that develop after birth.

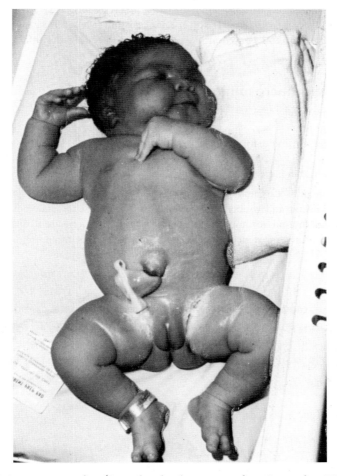

Figure 2-1. A macrosomic infant. (Reproduced with permission from Cunningham F, Leveno K, Bloom S, et al. *Williams Obstetrics,* 23rd ed. New York: McGraw-Hill; 2010).

What is the concern about macrosomia?

a. There are no complications
b. Hypoglycemia in the infant
c. Shoulder dystocia

d. Fetal adiposity
e. Pancreatic cancer as an adult

Answer c. Shoulder dystocia

Shoulder dystocia occurs when the infant's anterior shoulder gets stuck behind the pubic symphysis during childbirth (See Figure 7-19). Large infants are more likely to have a difficult labor complicated by shoulder dystocia. The larger the infant, the harder for the baby to come out and more likely to get stuck. Hypoglycemia in an infant after birth is a common complication that is easy to treat. Hypoglycemia in an infant develops because the fetus is used to a hyperglycemic environment in the mother. This causes an increase in the infant's circulating insulin. When born, the infant no longer has the large amounts of glucose in his or her system but still has high insulin levels. This causes the infant's blood sugar to drop and is a common complication. Feeding the infant resolves the hypoglycemia.

What causes macrosomia?

a. Thyroid hormone
b. Growth hormone
c. Insulin increases protein formation
d. Hyperlipidemia
e. Estrogen

Answer c. Insulin increases protein formation

The hyperglycemic state the infant is growing under leads to hyperplasia of β islet cells. This increases insulin and insulin-like growth factor. The other choices do not cause macrosomia, although thyroid hormone, estrogen, and growth hormone are all anabolic. Insulin is an anabolic hormone that increases the uptake of amino acids into protein.

Insulin works through tyrosine kinase receptor.
Continue to move the clock forward at the routine prenatal care pace: every 4 weeks until 28 weeks' gestation, every 2 weeks until 36 weeks' gestation, and weekly from 36 weeks' gestation until delivery. The patient's blood sugar remains controlled throughout the rest of the pregnancy.

CASE 3: HIV in Pregnancy

CC: *"I'm pregnant."*

Setting: *Outpatient office*

VS: *BP, 125/78 mm; P, 73 beats/min; R, 13 breaths/min; T, 98°F*

HPI: *A 28-year-old woman with no past medical history presents for her initial prenatal visit. Her last menstrual period (LMP) was 6 weeks ago.*

ROS:
- *Denies leakage of fluid*
- *Denies vaginal bleeding*
- *Denies fetal movement*
- *Denies contractions*
- *Nausea and vomiting present*

Labs:
- *Complete blood count (CBC): white blood cells (WBCs), 8 ×10³/μL; hemoglobin (Hgb), 11.0 g/dL; hematocrit (Hct), 33.5%; platelets, 167 ×10³/μL*
- *CMP: Sodium, 128 mmol/L; potassium, 4.5 mmol/L; chloride, 100 mmol/L; bicarbonate, 22 mmol/L; blood urea nitrogen (BUN), 0.9 mg/dL; creatinine, 1 mg/dL; glucose, 97 mg/dL*
- *Rubella IgG: positive*
- *HIV: positive*
- *CD4 count: 750*
- *Viral load: 20,000 copies/mL*
- *Hepatitis B sAg: Negative*
- *HgbA1c: 5.6%*

What drug is contraindicated in pregnancy?

a. Efavirenz

b. Nevirapine

c. Lopinavir

d. Ritonavir

e. Atazanavir

f. Zidovudine

Answer a. Efavirenz

Efavirenz is a non-nucleoside reverse transcriptase inhibitor (<u>NNRTI</u>) that is the first-line treatment in nonpregnant women. However, because of potential teratogenicity, it is not recommended in pregnant women. The rest of the drugs are acceptable during pregnancy. Zidovudine is considered a first-line treatment in pregnant women. Teratogenicity is not associated with any of the protease inhibitors

On the CCS, when a pregnant patient is HIV positive, the following should be ordered: HIV genotype, viral load, CD4 count, hepatitis panel, and treatment with highly active anti-retroviral therapy (HAART).

What is the next best step in the management of this patient?

a. Zidovudine now

b. Zidovudine starting in the second trimester

c. Zidovudine, lamivudine, ritonavir, and lopinavir now

d. Zidovudine, lamivudine, ritonavir, and lopinavir starting in the second trimester

Answer c. Zidovudine, lamivudine, ritonavir, and lopinavir now

Zidovudine, lamivudine, ritonavir, and lopinavir (HAART) should be started as soon as possible in pregnant patients. HAART has been shown to decrease maternal fetal transmission (i.e., vertical transmission) to less than 1%. Zidovudine has the best evidence for efficacy, so it should be included in any treatment combination. Overall, however, the efficacy of antiretrovirals in preventing the perinatal transmission of HIV is not as much related to a specific drug as it is to decreasing the viral load to an undetectable level.

Which of these tests is most useful in a pregnant woman to guide the use of therapy?

a. Genotyping

b. Polymerase chain reaction (PCR) RNA viral load

c. CD4

d. CBC

Answer a. Genotyping

Genotyping should be done in all HIV-positive persons at baseline to determine which therapy to give. Although PCR RNA viral load and CD4 cell count will be done, they are not as useful because all HIV-positive pregnant woman are treated at any CD4 and any viral load. Genotyping changes therapy. If the patient's virus is resistant to zidovudine or lamivudine, different therapy will be used. If, in an extreme circumstance, the patient's virus were resistant to all protease inhibitors and the only NNRTI that it was sensitive to was efavirenz, then efavirenz would be prescribed. Efficacy in preventing perinatal transmission is more important than adverse effects.

Genotyping drives the choice of the right therapy.

Monotherapy is not used in any HIV-positive person for any reason.

Move the clock forward to the 14-week prenatal visit.

Interval History: *The patient is feeling well. She continues her HIV medications, which include zidovudine, lamivudine, and lopinavir/ritonavir.*

What is the next step in the management of this patient?

a. Amniocentesis

b. Chest radiography

c. Hepatitis C serologic testing

d. Toxoplasmosis titers

Answer c. Hepatitis C serologic testing

Hepatitis B and C testing should be done on all patients with HIV. There is a high co-infectivity rate secondary to the shared routes of transmission. Amniocentesis should be avoided in HIV-positive patients with a high viral load. All invasive procedures should be avoided if possible. Chest radiography and toxoplasmosis titers are not routinely recommended in pregnant patients with HIV. PPD or interferon-γ release assay is indicated. Although the perinatal transmission of hepatitis C is extremely small, all HIV-positive persons should be tested. There is no specific therapy for the infant even if the mother is hepatitis C seropositive. Ninety percent of those who got HIV through injection drug use are also seropositive for hepatitis C.

If the patient were to be purified protein derivative (PPD) skin test positive, what is the right management?

a. No further action is needed.

b. Give isoniazid for 9 months.

c. Do chest radiography; if findings are negative, give isoniazid for 9 months.

d. Check sputum acid-fast stains.

e. Do chest radiography; if findings are negative, no further action is needed.

Answer c. Do chest radiography; if findings are negative, give isoniazid for 9 months.

Do chest radiography; if findings are negative, isoniazid should be given for 9 months. PPD skin testing and interferon-γ release assay (IGRA) tell who is at risk for latent tuberculosis (TB) infection. Doing one of these tests is particularly important in HIV-positive persons. In the general population, the risk of TB with a reactive test is only 10% in a lifetime. In those with HIV, it can be as high as 10% a year.

If the PPD or IGRA result is positive, chest radiography must be done even if the mother is HIV positive. A lead shield should be placed over the patient's abdomen to do the radiograph. Even if the radiographic findings are negative, you must give isoniazid during pregnancy. Isoniazid is not teratogenic. It is especially important to give it to HIV-positive pregnant women because of the high risk of reactivation of TB in those with HIV. HIV-positive women need isoniazid during pregnancy. If the immune system is normal, treatment can wait until after delivery.

> Do PPD in every HIV-positive mother. If the result is positive (>5 mm), do chest radiography and give isoniazid for 9 months.

> Move the clock forward to 36 weeks' gestation.
>
> **Setting:** Outpatient office
>
> **Interval History:** The patient is feeling well and continues to take her medications. She denies any complaints.
>
> **Labs:**
> - CD 4 count: 500
> - Viral load: 500 copies/mL

How and when should the patient deliver the infant?

a. At 39 weeks' gestation via C-section
b. At 40 weeks' gestation via C-section
c. Spontaneous vaginal delivery

d. Induction at 39 weeks' gestation for vaginal delivery

Answer c. Spontaneous vaginal delivery

Patients with a viral load less than 1000 copies/mL can deliver via the vaginal route. Patients who have a viral load less than 1000 copies/mL have very low rates of transmission. However, if the patient has a viral load of more than 1000 copies/mL at 38 weeks' gestation, a C-section should be scheduled for 39 weeks' gestation. Invasive testing during labor, such as scalp electrodes, should be avoided. Perinatal transmission rate with full viral suppression to undetectable or nearly undetectable viral load levels is less than 2%.

> Move the clock forward to after delivery.
>
> **Interval History:** The patient delivered a baby boy born via normal spontaneous vaginal delivery at 39 weeks' gestation. The delivery was uncomplicated.

What is the next step in the management of this patient?

a. The patient should breastfeed her infant.
b. Start the newborn on zidovudine, lamivudine, ritonavir, and lopinavir.
c. Start the newborn on zidovudine.

d. Formula the feed newborn with no drug therapy.
e. Give zidovudine and HIV immune globulin.

Answer c. Start the newborn on zidovudine.

Newborns of HIV-positive mothers must not be breastfed. There is an increased risk of vertical transmission through breastfeeding. All newborns of HIV-positive mothers should receive 6 weeks of zidovudine starting within 12 hours of delivery. The mother should receive intrapartum intravenous zidovudine. HIV-specific immune globulin was disproven to help prevent perinatal HIV transmission some time ago. It is never correct.

Breastfeeding by an HIV-positive mother is child abuse.

What is the most common adverse effect of zidovudine?

a. Peripheral neuropathy
b. Pancreatitis
c. Hyperlipidemia

d. Macrocytic anemia
e. Megaloblastic anemia

Answer d. Macrocytic anemia

Zidovudine causes an increase in mean corpuscular volume (MCV). There is no hypersegmentation of neutrophils. Macrocytosis means an increased MCV (Figure 2-2). Megaloblastic means hypersegmentation of neutrophils. Peripheral neuropathy and pancreatitis are caused by stavudine and didanosine. Hyperlipidemia is an adverse effect of protease inhibitors.

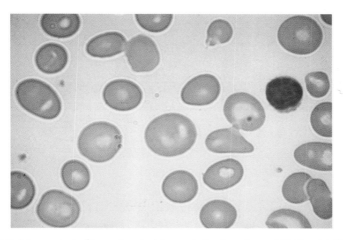

Figure 2-2. Macrocytosis. (Reproduced with permission from Longo DL, Fauci A, Kasper D, et al. *Harrison's Principles of Internal Medicine*, 18th ed, vol. 1. New York: McGraw-Hill; 2012.)

Macrocytosis = Large red blood cells
Megaloblastic = Hypersegmentation of neutrophils

Zidovudine inhibits reverse transcriptase.
Reverse transcriptase converts RNA into DNA.

Move the clock forward 2 weeks.

Which of the following tests is best to use to exclude HIV infection in an infant?

a. HIV antibody test

b. HIV DNA PCR

c. p24 antigen

d. Viral culture

Answer b. HIV DNA PCR

The diagnosis of HIV in infants of HIV-positive mothers is the only time to use the HIV DNA PCR of peripheral blood mononuclear cells. The HIV antibody test is unreliable in infants.

CASE 4: Peripartum Cardiomyopathy

CC: *"I can't breathe."*

Setting: *Outpatient office*

VS: *BP, 135/80 mm Hg; P, 78 beats/min; R, 26 breaths/min; T, 98.6°F*

HPI: *A 36-year-old G_3P_{2002} with an IUP at 38 weeks presents for shortness of breath. Shortness of breath has been gradually getting worse for the past 2 weeks. The patient states that she now needs to sleep with three pillows to feel like she can breathe.*

ROS:
- *Chest pain: Negative*
- *Cough: Negative*
- *Hemoptysis: Negative*
- *Fever: Negative*
- *Edema: Positive*
- *Fetal movement: Positive*
- *Contractions: Negative*
- *Vaginal bleeding: Negative*
- *Leakage of fluid: Negative*

Physical Exam
- *Cardiovascular system (CVS): S_1S_2 + Regular Rate and Rhythm (RRR) no murmurs*
- *Lungs: + Crackles bilaterally*
- *Abd: gravid*
- *Ext: 2+ edema bilaterally*

What is the next best step in the management of this patient?

a. CBC

b. CMP

c. Brain natriuretic peptide (BNP)

d. Chest computed tomography (CT)

Answer c. Brain natriuretic peptide (BNP)

The patient is complaining of symptoms of heart failure. She has shortness of breath and orthopnea that is worsening. Although peripheral edema is normal in pregnant women, if it is coupled of other symptoms than congestive heart failure should be considered. BNP is elevated in patients with heart failure. If the BNP finding is negative, it will exclude the possibility of peripartum cardiomyopathy. CBC and CMP will not help exclude causes of chest pain. Radiation exposure is avoided as much as possible in pregnant women. If the diagnosis cannot be made without the chest radiography, fetal and abdominal shielding should be used. Chest radiography, not chest CT, would be the first-line imaging. In this case, the blood tests should be done first.

On the CCS, the initial order set should include CBC, CMP, BNP, chest radiography with fetal and abdominal shield, D-dimer, arterial blood gas (ABG) analysis, and electrocardiography (ECG). These test results will help guide you to a more likely differential diagnosis.

> BNP normal function:
> • Stretch of atrium increases level
> • Increases urinary loss of sodium and water
> On the CCS, do not forget to move the patient to the labor and delivery or inpatient unit after the initial order set is placed.

Move the clock forward to the next available laboratory test result.

Setting: *Labor and delivery (inpatient)*

- *CBC: WBC, 5.8 ×10³/μL; Hgb, 11.5 g/dL; Hct, 33%; platelets, 200 ×10³/μL*
- *CMP: Sodium, 126 mmol/L; potassium, 4.2 mmol/L; chloride, 110 mmol/L; bicarbonate, 22 mmol/L; BUN, 0.8 mg/dL; creatinine, 1 mg/dL; glucose, 115 mg/dL*
- *BNP: 10,000 (markedly elevated)*

Which test is the most specific?

a. ECG
b. Echocardiography
c. BNP

d. Cardiac magnetic resonance imaging (MRI)

Answer b. Echocardiography

The last laboratory test results show that the patient has an elevated BNP, which is indicative of heart failure. Echocardiography is the most specific test to show the ejection fraction (EF). ECG findings may be abnormal but will not quantify the severity of the heart failure. ECG may indicate the cause, such as acute myocardial infarction. BNP is sensitive but not specific. Cardiac MRI is controversial to use in pregnancy and in congestive heart failure (CHF) in general. The cardiac MRI has not found a clear place in clinical management at this time.

On the CCS, both the ECG and echocardiography should be ordered. Normal BNP excludes CHF. Elevated BNP is nonspecific.

> *Move the clock forward to the next available laboratory test result.*
>
> **Interval History:**
> • *ECG: Sinus tachycardia; no other abnormalities*
> • *Echocardiogram: EF 35%*
> • *Chest radiography: Mild enlargement of the heart and pulmonary congestion visualized*

Which medication should be given at this time?

a. Coumadin
b. Dobutamine
c. Furosemide

d. Lisinopril
e. Digoxin

Answer **c.** Furosemide

The patient has shortness of breath. The treatment for shortness of breath that is secondary to pulmonary edema is furosemide. It is a class C drug. However, because the mother has pulmonary edema, the benefits outweigh the risks. Relieving hypoxia and dyspnea from fluid overload is more beneficial than the possible shunting of blood away from the placenta. The fetus cannot do well if the mother has hypoxia. Coumadin is a class X drug that is contraindicated in pregnancy. Dobutamine may be given in pregnancy, but it would not be used first. Dobutamine is used in acute pulmonary edema for those not responding to preload reduction with diuretics, morphine, and nitrates. Dobutamine has no net effect on BP. Digoxin may be given in pregnancy, but it is not a first-line therapy for heart failure in any patient. Lisinopril, as well as any ACE inhibitor or angiotensin receptor blocker, is contraindicated in pregnancy. If this patient was not pregnant, it would be a first-line treatment for CHF.

What is the mechanism of dobutamine in acute pulmonary edema?

a. Positive inotrope
b. Positive inotrope and afterload reduction

c. Preload reduction
d. Preload reduction and positive inotrope

Answer **b.** Positive inotrope and afterload reduction

Dobutamine and dopamine are both positive inotropes that increase the contractility of the heart. The main difference between them is that dopamine has an α-agonist effect that increases afterload. Dobutamine is a peripheral vasodilator. This is why there is no net effect on BP. Dobutamine increases contractility, which increases cardiac output, but the vasodilatory effect results in no net effect on BP. More blood is ejected into a bigger potential space.

Move the clock forward 2 weeks.

Interval History: *The patient is feeling better. Labor was induced, and the patient gave birth to a healthy baby boy.*

What is the recommendation for after the pregnancy?

a. As long as the patient is stable on medications, she may have another child.

b. The patient should not have another child.

c. The patient should wait 2 or 3 years before trying to have another baby.

d. There are no restrictions or treatment. She may have another child at any time.

Answer b. The patient should not have another child.

Peripartum cardiomyopathy holds significant risks to both the mother and fetus of subsequent pregnancies. Patients with persistent left ventricular (LV) dysfunction should avoid pregnancy. The pregnancy recommendations for patients with recovered LV function are still controversial, but they will have a decline in LV function during the pregnancy.

CASE 5: Pulmonary Embolism in Pregnancy

CC: *"I'm short of breath."*

Setting: *Emergency department*

VS: *BP, 120/80 mm Hg; P, 120 beats/min; R, 24 breaths/min; T, 98.9°F; pulse ox, 89% on room air*

HPI: *A 28-year-old G_1P_0 with an IUP at 26 weeks' gestation presents to the emergency department for shortness of breath. She receives regular prenatal care, and her pregnancy has been uncomplicated thus far. She developed shortness of breath suddenly after a long drive in traffic. She has chest pain when she takes a deep breath.*

PE:
- *General: awake, alert, oriented ×3, mild respiratory distress*
- *CVS: S_1S_2+ RRR no m/r/g*
- *Lungs: Clear to auscultation bilaterally*
- *Abd: Gravid; fundal height 25 cm; no tenderness*
- *Ext: 1+ edema bilaterally; no erythema*
- *Chest radiography with an abdominal shield is within normal limits.*

What is the next best step?

a. CBC

b. CMP

c. D-Dimer

d. Doppler ultrasonography of the legs

Answer d. Doppler ultrasonography of the legs

This patient presents with a sudden onset of shortness of breath, tachycardia, and low oxygen saturation. This combination is suspicious for pulmonary embolism (PE). PE evaluation in a *nonpregnant* person begins with a D-dimer. D-Dimer is a very sensitive test for PE. However, in pregnant patients, the D-dimer is often elevated and no longer sensitive. About 80% of pregnant women in the second trimester have elevated D-dimers. CBC and CMP will not help rule in or out the diagnosis. ABG analysis is not done in pregnant patients because respiratory alkalosis is very common in pregnant women regardless of whether there is a PE. Doppler ultrasonography of the legs is often used to verify the presence of deep vein thrombosis (DVT). If a DVT is present, the treatment is the same as for a PE, and no further testing is necessary. Ultrasonography is a safe test in pregnancy, and the fetus would not be exposed to any radiation. Therefore, Doppler ultrasonography is the first-line test in this pregnant patient with leg swelling.

On the CCS, the following should be included in the initial order set: CBC, CMP, D-dimer, chest radiography with abdominal shielding, ABG, Doppler ultrasonography of bilateral lower extremities, and oxygen via nasal canula. PT , PTT, INR

ABG

D-Dimer is a fibrin degradation product.

Virchow's triad = Stasis, endothelial injury, and hypercoagulability

Plasmin breaks up fibrin into D-dimers.

Move the clock forward to the next available laboratory test result.

Interval History: *The patient continues to feel short of breath. Oxygen via nasal cannula has been given. Doppler ultrasonography findings of the bilateral lower extremities are negative.*

What is the next step in the management?

a. CT angiography of the chest

b. Chest radiography

c. MRI of the chest

d. Ventilation/perfusion (V/Q) scan

Answer d. Ventilation/perfusion (V/Q) scan

V/Q scan the next step in the management of pregnant women with possible PE. V/Q scan has less radiation to both the mother and fetus compared with chest CT or CT angiography. If the chest radiography showed some abnormalities, then the next step would have been CT angiography. MRI of the chest is controversial at this time. Chest radiography was already done, and repeating it would not yield any more information.

Move the clock forward to the next available laboratory test result.

Interval History: *The V/Q scan is positive for PE.*

What is the treatment of choice?

a. Warfarin

b. Intravenous unfractionated heparin

c. Subcutaneous unfractionated heparin

d. Low-molecular-weight heparin (LMWH)

Answer d. Low-molecular-weight heparin (LMWH)

LMWH is recommended over both intravenous and subcutaneous unfractionated heparin secondary to its ease of use and safety profile. Warfarin is contraindicated in pregnancy.

Treatment should be continued throughout the pregnancy. LMWH should be discontinued 24 hours before any planned delivery (i.e., induction or C-section).

> *Move the clock forward every 2 weeks until 36 weeks' gestation.*
>
> **Setting:** *Outpatient office*
>
> **Interval History:** *The patient continues to take enoxaparin, and no complications are noted. Routine prenatal care continues.*
>
> *Move the clock forward weekly until 39 weeks' gestation.*
>
> **Interval History:** *The patient gave birth via elective C-section at 39 weeks' gestation. LMWH was stopped 24 hours before delivery. There were no complications during delivery, and no significant bleeding occurred.*

What is the next step in the management of this patient?

a. Restart LMWH 12 hours after delivery.
b. Restart LMWH 24 hours after delivery.
c. Start warfarin 24 hours after delivery.
d. Place an inferior vena cava filter.

Answer b. Restart LMWH 24 hours after delivery.

Anticoagulation should be restarted 24 hours after a C-section or 6 hours after a vaginal delivery. The anticoagulant of choice is LMWH. Bridging therapy with warfarin may be started after 24 hours of LMWH. Concomitant therapy with warfarin and LMWH should occur for 5 days or until the international normalized ratio (INR) is therapeutic (between 2 and 3). Warfarin is considered safe during lactation. Warfarin should continue for 6 months after a PE or DVT. A vena cava filter is used in those with a contraindication to anticoagulation.

> Warfarin is contraindicated during pregnancy but safe during lactation.

> Warfarin inhibits factors II, VII, IX, and X (Figure 2-3).

What is one of the long-term side effects of prolonged use of LMWH?

a. Bleeding
b. Thrombocytopenia
c. Skin necrosis
d. Osteoporosis

Answer d. Osteoporosis

Patients who undergo LMWH for more than 7 weeks are at increased risk for osteoporosis. Bleeding, thrombocytopenia, and skin necrosis are complications that arise while taking

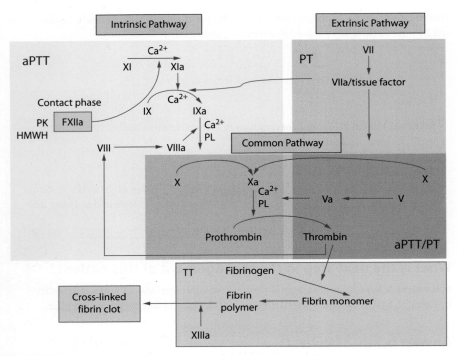

Figure 2-3. Clotting cascade and the laboratory test results that are affected. aPTT, activated partial thromboplastin time; PT, prothrombin time; TT, thrombin time. (Reproduced with permission from Longo DL, Fauci A, Kasper D, et al. *Harrison's Principles of Internal Medicine*, 18th ed, vol. 1. New York: McGraw-Hill; 2012).

the medication. The mechanism of the osteoporosis in LMWH is not clear, but LMWH does appear to alter osteoblastic and osteoclastic function.

Heparin potentiates antithrombin.
Antithrombin inhibits almost all steps in clotting cascade.

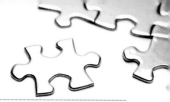

CHAPTER 3

VAGINAL BLEEDING

CASE 1: Induced Abortion

CC: *"I'm pregnant but don't want to have a baby."*

Setting: *Outpatient clinic*

VS: *BP, 115/75 mm Hg; P, 78 beats/min; R, 20 breaths/min; T, 98.6°F*

HPI: *A 21-year-old woman G_1P_0 with an intrauterine pregnancy (IUP) at 8 weeks' gestation presents for her first prenatal visit. The patient states that she would like to have a termination of the pregnancy. She denies any medical history, surgical history, allergies, and taking any medications.*

ROS:
- *Fetal movement: Negative*
- *Contractions: Negative*
- *Vaginal bleeding: Negative*
- *Leakage of fluid: Negative*

What laboratory studies need to be done before consideration of this request?

a. CMP

b. Blood type and screen

c. UA

d. HIV

e. Rapid plasma reagin (RPR)

Answer b. Blood type and screen

Pregnant patients should receive all of the above tests; however, the blood type and screen is particularly important in possible elective abortions. If the patient is known to be Rh negative, then RhoGAM should be given at the time of the abortion. This is because Rh-positive blood from the fetus may leak into maternal blood at the time of the termination. This would promote the development of antibodies against the minor blood group antigen Rh. You are doing the type and cross because an Rh-positive mother would not need RhoGAM, but an Rh-negative mother would need it.

On the CCS, initial order sets should include a complete blood count (CBC), comprehensive metabolic panel (CMP), HIV, blood type and screen, and transvaginal ultrasonography (US).

Move the clock forward 1 week.

Interval History:
- CBC: White blood cells (WBCs), 5.4 × 10³/μL; hemoglobin (Hgb), 12.0 g/dL; hematocrit (Hct), 36%; platelets, 215 × 10³/μL
- CMP: Sodium, 125 mmol/L; potassium, 4.3 mmol/L; chloride, 98 mmol/L; bicarbonate, 22 mmol/L; blood urea nitrogen (BUN), 9 mg/dL; creatinine, 0.8 mg/dL; glucose, 102 mg/dL; blood type, O+
- HIV: Negative
- RPR: Nonreactive

What is the best option for elective abortion?

a. Wait until after 15 weeks' gestation for dilation and evacuation

b. Start methotrexate now

c. Dilation and evacuation now

Answer c. Dilation and evacuation now

Elective terminations should be done as early as possible. The later in gestation the abortion occurs, the more difficult the procedure. It is always preferable to perform termination in the first trimester. Patients may elect for surgical or medical termination. Medical termination consists of methotrexate and misoprostol together or just misoprostol alone.

What is misoprostol?

a. A rigid dilator
b. An osmotic dilator
c. A prostaglandin E1 analog
d. An antiprogesterone
e. A prostacyclin analog

Answer c. A prostaglandin E1 analog

Misoprostol is a prostaglandin E1 analog that causes a cervical ripening, allowing the cervix to become softer and start to dilate. Rigid dilators are mechanical dilators that are used during surgical procedures that forcefully dilate the cervix. Osmotic dilators are used to soften the cervix, similar to the prostaglandin E1 analogs. Examples of osmotic dilators are seaweed and Lamicel. Mifepristone is an antiprogesterone that promotes cervical dilation; however, it is not recommended. The prostacyclin analogues are epoprostenol, treprostinil, and iloprost. They are used in pulmonary hypertension.

Do you have to perform elective abortions?

a. Yes, under all circumstances
b. Yes, if it is in the first trimester
c. Yes, if it is an emergency
d. No

Answer d. No

The physician is not required to perform elective abortions. Some physicians choose to provide this service. If a patient of yours would like to have this done and you do not perform this service, you should refer the patient to another physician. If the situation arises when there is an emergency need for a dilation and evacuation, this is no longer "elective." You are never required to perform an elective procedure that you have an ethical objection to. In the case of an emergency or unstable patient, you must make sure the service is provided, but it does not have to be by you.

Ethical and legal questions must have a correct answer that is valid in all 50 states.

Move the clock forward 1 week.

Interval History: *The patient had a successful medical termination of pregnancy.*

CASE 2: Spontaneous Abortion

CC: *"I'm pregnant and have vaginal bleeding."*

Setting: *Emergency department*

VS: *BP, 120/80 mm Hg; P, 76 beats/min; R, 12 breaths/min; T, 98.6°F*

HPI: *A 29-year-old G_2P_{1001} with an IUP at 7 weeks' gestation presents to the emergency department (ED) for vaginal bleeding. She started to have abdominal pain and vaginal bleeding overnight. No clots were expressed per the vagina. She denies any other medical history, surgical history, and allergies. The patient is taking prenatal vitamins. The bleeding started after sexual relations.*

ROS:
- *Fetal movement: Negative*
- *Contractions: Unsure what the abdominal pain is*
- *Vaginal bleeding: Positive*
- *Leakage of fluid: Negative*

PE:
- *CVS: Normal*
- *Lungs: Normal*
- *Abd: Soft, nontender, nondistended, +BS*
- *Ext: No edema*
- *Sterile speculum exam: Cervix closed; blood in vaginal vault*

What is the next step?

a. Abdominal US
b. Beta-human chorionic gonadotropin (BHCG)
c. Computed tomography (CT) scan
d. RhoGAM
e. Discharge home with follow-up as an outpatient

Answer b. Beta-human chorionic gonadotropin (BHCG)

On the CCS, the following should be ordered after doing the history and physical examination: CBC, blood type and screen, BHCG, and transvaginal US. As a single best answer, BHCG is done to ensure that the patient was pregnant and to have a baseline. The BHCG level should double every 48 hours if the pregnancy is developing normally. At a BHCG level of 1000 to 1500 mlU/L is an indication that a gestational sac should be seen on US. In early pregnancy, transvaginal US is more sensitive and specific than transabdominal US. A CT scan will expose the fetus to radiation and should be avoided if possible during pregnancy. RhoGAM may need to be given. Blood type and screen needs to be done first. You do not have to give RhoGAM to Rh-positive mothers. Discharging the patient home without laboratory examination or US is inappropriate. You need to be sure the fetus is viable and there has not been significant blood loss.

> On the CCS, the following should be ordered initially: CBC, blood type and screen, BHCG, and transvaginal US.
>
> Move the clock forward to the next available test results.
>
> **Interval History:**
> - CBC: WBC, $6.3 \times 10^3/\mu L$; Hgb, 11.1 g/dL; Hct, 33.9%; platelets, $250 \times 10^3/\mu L$
> - CMP: Sodium, 125 mmol/L; potassium, 4.2 mmol/L; chloride, 98 mmol/L; bicarbonate, 21 mmol/L; BUN, 8 mg/dL; creatinine, 0.5 mg/dL; glucose, 97 mg/dL
> - Blood type: AB+
> - Transvaginal US results: Cervix open; products of conception seen; intrauterine bleeding

What is the most likely diagnosis?

a. Complete abortion
b. Incomplete abortion
c. Inevitable abortion

d. Threatened abortion
e. Missed abortion
f. Septic abortion

Answer c. Inevitable abortion

US is the only way to distinguish between the different types of abortions. Complete abortion means that all of the products of conception have been expelled and the cervix is closed (Figure 3-1). Incomplete abortion means that some products of conception are left behind but the cervix is still closed (Figure 3-2). Inevitable abortion occurs when there are productions of conception but the cervix is open and intrauterine bleeding is seen. Threatened abortion occurs when there are products of conception and intrauterine bleeding but a closed cervix. Missed abortion occurs when there is no fetal heart beat seen and all the products of conception are present. Septic abortion is defined as an infection of the uterus and the surrounding areas.

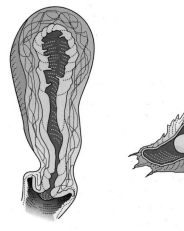

Figure 3-1. Complete abortion. (Reproduced with permission from Benson RC. *Handbook of Obstetrics & Gynecology*, 9th ed. New York: Lange/McGraw-Hill; 1994.)

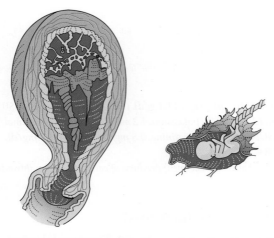

Figure 3-2. Incomplete abortion. (Reproduced with permission from Benson RC. *Handbook of Obstetrics & Gynecology,* 9th ed. New York: Lange/McGraw-Hill; 1994.)

Type	US Finding	Treatment
Complete	No products of conception; cervix closed	Follow-up BHCG in office
Incomplete	Some products of conception found; cervix closed	Dilation and curettage (D&C)
Inevitable	Products of conception present; intrauterine bleeding; dilation of cervix	Medical induction or D&C
Threatened	Products of conception found; intrauterine bleeding; no dilation of cervix	Bed rest
Missed	Death of fetus but still in the uterus	Medical induction or D&C
Septic	Infection of the uterus	D&C and intravenous levofloxacin and metronidazole

What is the treatment of choice?

a. D&C

b. Methotrexate

c. Follow-up in the office

d. Repeat BHCG in 2 days

e. Intravenous (IV) levofloxacin

Answer a. D&C

Treatment of incomplete abortion, inevitable abortion, and missed abortion are the same. They can be treated either medically or surgically. Medical management with misoprostol will ripen the cervix and begin contractions. Surgically, a D&C will manually remove the productions of conception. Patients with complete abortion will need follow-up in the office, and the BHCG level should be followed until it returns to zero. Threatened abortions are still viable fetuses. The mother should be placed on pelvic rest. Septic abortions are treated with IV metronidazole and IV levofloxacin.

What is the most common reason for spontaneous abortion?

a. Anatomic abnormality

b. Chromosomal abnormality

c. Diabetes

d. Sexually transmitted infections

e. Trauma

Answer b. Chromosomal abnormality

All of these are causes of spontaneous abortions. However, the most common cause is chromosomal abnormalities, accounting for 60% to 80% of spontaneous abortions. Most spontaneous abortions occur before 12 weeks of gestation.

Spontaneous abortion = Before 20 weeks' gestation
Fetal demise = After 20 weeks' gestation

Move the clock forward 1 week.

Interval History: *The patient had a D&C 1 week ago. The patient denies abdominal pain and vaginal bleeding. The patient is doing well.*

CASE 3: Placenta Previa

CC: *"I'm pregnant and have vaginal bleeding."*

Setting: *Emergency department*

VS: *BP, 110/80 mm Hg; P, 95 beats/min; R, 12 breaths/min; T, 98.6°F*

HPI: *A 29-year-old G_2P_{1001} with an IUP at 35 weeks' gestation presents to the ED for vaginal bleeding. The patient states that she woke up in a puddle of blood. She denies abdominal pain. She also denies other medical history, surgical history, and allergies. The patient is taking prenatal vitamins.*

ROS:
- *Fetal movement: Present*
- *Contractions: Absent*
- *Vaginal bleeding: Present*
- *Leakage of fluid: Absent*

PE:
- *CVS: Normal*
- *Lungs: Clear bilaterally*
- *Abd: Gravid, nontender, nondistended, +BS*
- *Ext: No edema bilaterally*

What is the next step in the management of this patient?

a. Transvaginal US

b. Digital vaginal examination

c. Abdominal US

d. Fetal fibronectin level

Answer c. Abdominal US

This patient is experiencing third trimester *painless* vaginal bleeding. This is placenta previa until proven otherwise. Placenta previa is defined as the placenta covering the internal os of the cervix. There are three types: complete, partial, and marginal. If digital examination is done, the fingers passing through the cervix may cause worsening of the vaginal bleeding by further separating the placenta from the uterus. This is the same for a transvaginal US. Fetal fibronectin is not done at 35 weeks. Fetal fibronectin is done between 22 and 34 weeks of gestational age when preterm labor is being considered. A transabdominal US should be done first to locate the placenta.

Fibronectin is "placenta glue."

Complete placenta previa = Placenta *completely* covers the internal os (Figure 3-3)

Partial placenta previa = Placenta *partially* covers the internal os (Figure 3-4)

Marginal placenta previa = Placenta is *near* the internal os (Figure 3-5)

Vasa previa = Fetal vessels (umbilical cord) cover the internal os

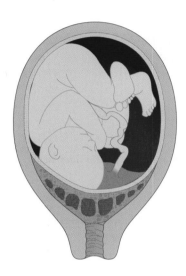

Figure 3-3. Complete placenta previa. (Reproduced with permission from Tintinalli JE, Stapczynski J, Ma OJ, et al. *Tintinalli's Emergency Medicine: A Comprehensive Study Guide*, 7th ed. New York: McGraw-Hill; 2011.)

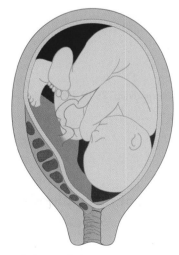

Figure 3-4. Partial placenta previa. (Reproduced with permission from Tintinalli JE, Stapczynski J, Ma OJ, et al. *Tintinalli's Emergency Medicine: A Comprehensive Study Guide*, 7th ed. New York: McGraw-Hill; 2011.)

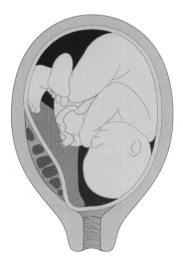

Figure 3-5. Marginal placental previa. (Reproduced with permission from Tintinalli JE, Stapczynski J, Ma OJ, et al. *Tintinalli's Emergency Medicine: A Comprehensive Study Guide*, 7th ed. New York: McGraw-Hill; 2011.)

On CCS, the following orders should be written after the initial history: CBC, type and screen, prothrombin time (PT), partial thromboplastin time (PTT), international normalized ratio (INR), transabdominal US, fetal monitoring, and maternal cardiac monitoring.

If placental abnormalities are being considered, transfer the patient to the inpatient unit!

NEVER do a digital vaginal or transvaginal US in PAINLESS vaginal bleeding in the third trimester!

Move the clock forward 1 hour.
Transfer the patient to the inpatient unit.

Interval History: *The patient's vaginal bleeding has stopped. The patient continues to feel fetal movement.*

Maternal Heart Monitor: *Normal sinus rhythm*

Fetal Heart Tracing: *Reactive, accelerations are present, no decelerations, good variability*

Greater variability in heart rate = More life in fetuses

Labs:
- *CBC: WBC, 5 × 10³/µL; Hgb, 10.5 g/dL; Hct, 31%; platelets, 250 × 10³/µL*
- *Blood type: O+*
- *INR: 1.0*

Transabdominal US: Partial placenta previa

What is the next step in the management of this patient?

a. Immediate C-section
b. Immediate induction of labor
c. Bed rest
d. Transfuse 2 units of packed red cells (PRBCs)
e. Administer betamethasone

Answer c. Bed rest

Treatment conservatively at this point is the best option. The vaginal bleeding has stopped, and both the mother and fetus are fine. The patient does not have a significant drop in Hgb or

Hct. The patient should undergo pelvic rest (meaning nothing per the vagina, including intercourse) for the rest of her pregnancy. Delivery by either modality is premature because both the mother and fetus are doing well. If either was hemodynamically unstable, a cesarean section (C-section) would be necessary. The patient should plan to have an elective C-section. Transfusion of PRBCs is not indicated at this time. All pregnant women are anemic, often to this level; oral ferrous sulfate should be administered. Betamethasone should be given if delivery is being considered in women from 23 to 34 weeks of gestation. Betamethasone will help mature fetal lungs and decrease the incidence of respiratory disease of the newborn.

Indications for immediate C-section:
- Severe hemorrhage
- Fetal distress
- Cervical dilation more than 4 cm

VAGINAL delivery is NOT indicated in placenta previa.

Placenta previa, even if resolved, is a risk factor for vasa previa.
Vasa previa is defined at the fetal or umbilical vessels lying in front of the internal cervical os.

Vasa previa:
- May be seen on transvaginal US (Figure 3-6)
- May be felt on digital cervical examination
- If not diagnosed before labor, will present as vaginal bleeding after rupture of membranes with fetal heart abnormalities
- Fetal blood loss with rapid exsanguination and fetal death

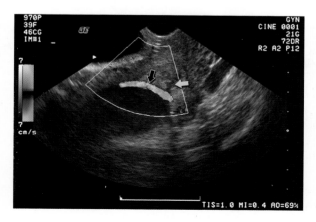

Figure 3-6. Ultrasound showing vasa previa. (Reproduced with permission from Cunningham F, Leveno K, Bloom S, et al. *Williams Obstetrics,* 23rd ed. New York: McGraw-Hill; 2010.)

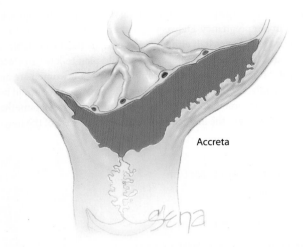

Figure 3-7. Placenta accreta. (Reproduced with permission from Cunningham F, Leveno K, Bloom S, et al. *Williams Obstetrics,* 23rd ed. New York: McGraw-Hill; 2010.)

Placental invasion is associated with placenta previa.
- Diagnosed when placenta cannot detach from the uterine walls
  - Placenta accreta: Invasion into the superficial uterine wall (Figure 3-7)
  - Placenta increta: Invasion into the uterine myometrium (Figure 3-8)
  - Placenta percreta: Invasion into the uterine serosa, bladder wall, or rectal wall (Figure 3-9)

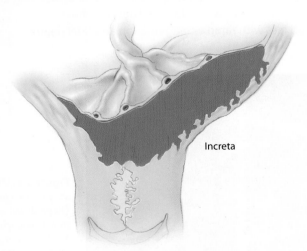

Figure 3-8. Placenta increta. (Reproduced with permission from Cunningham F, Leveno K, Bloom S, et al. *Williams Obstetrics,* 23rd ed. New York: McGraw-Hill; 2010.)

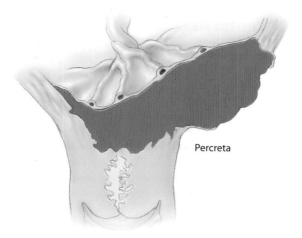

Percreta

Figure 3-9. Placenta percreta. (Reproduced with permission from Cunningham F, Leveno K, Bloom S, et al. *Williams Obstetrics,* 23rd ed. New York: McGraw-Hill; 2010.)

Move the clock forward 1 week.

The patient has continued on bed rest without any other complications. The patient will continue prenatal care and bed rest until delivery.

CASE 4: Placental Abruption

CC: *"I'm pregnant have vaginal bleeding and abdominal pain."*

Setting: *Emergency department*

VS: *BP, 110/80 mm Hg; P, 95 beats/min; R, 12 breaths/min; T, 98.6°F*

HPI: *A 29-year-old G_2P_{1001} with an IUP at 35 weeks' gestation presents to the ED for vaginal bleeding. The patient states that she was at work when she suddenly felt a sharp abdominal pain. The abdominal pain is worsening. She denies other medical history, surgical history, and allergies. The patient is taking prenatal vitamins. The patient is a known cocaine user.*

ROS:
- *Fetal movement: Present*
- *Contractions: Unsure what the abdominal pain is*
- *Vaginal bleeding: Present*
- *Leakage of fluid: Absent*

PE:
- *CVS: Normal*
- *Lungs: Clear bilaterally*
- *Abd: Gravid, nontender, nondistended, +BS*
- *Ext: No edema bilaterally*

What is the next step in the management of this patient?

a. Abdominal US

b. Transvaginal US

c. Digital cervical examination

d. Fetal fibronectin level

e. HIV test

Answer c. Digital cervical examination

This patient may be experiencing some signs of normal labor (i.e., contractions). However, with her history of cocaine abuse, abruption placenta should be ruled out. The first step in patients who are in their third trimester with abdominal pain and vaginal bleeding is to do a digital cervical examination. If the cervix is dilated, then the patient is in labor. If the cervix is not dilated, then an abdominal US to visualize the placenta is done. Transvaginal US may not visualize the entire placenta. HIV testing and fetal fibronectin level would not help determine a diagnosis at this point.

On the CCS, the initial order set should include physical exam (including digital cervical examination), CBC, CMP, blood type and screen, PT, PTT, INR, fibrinogen, maternal and fetal monitoring, IV fluids, and maternal oxygen.

If placental abnormalities are being considered, then transfer the patient to the inpatient unit!

Placenta previa = *Painless* vaginal bleeding = *No* cervical examination

Abruptio placenta = *Painful* vaginal bleeding = Cervical examination

---

What is placental abruption?

a. Placental hypercontractability

b. Placental insufficiency

c. Premature placental separation

d. Placental thrombosis

Answer c. Premature placental separation

Placental abruption is defined as partial or complete separation of placenta from the uterus before delivery of the fetus. It is the separation of the decidua basalis from the anchoring villi of the placenta. The detached portion cannot exchange gasses or nutrients.

Which risk factor is modifiable?

a. Trauma

b. Hypertension

c. Smoking

d. Eclampsia

Answer c. Smoking

Smoking is one of the only modifiable risk factors. That is, when the patient quits smoking, the risk of abruption decreases. Patients who smoke have more than double the risk for abruption causing fetal death. This risk increases even more if they have hypertension as well. The risk increases by 40% for each pack smoked per day. Hypertension causes a fivefold increase in risk of abruption, but even when controlled with medication, the risk does not seem to decrease. Treatment of eclampsia is delivery; therefore, it does not modify the risk of abruption.

Risk factors for placental abruption:
• Smoking
• Trauma
• Cocaine use
• Hypertension
• Preeclampsia or eclampsia

Move the clock forward to the next available results.

Setting: *Inpatient unit (labor and delivery)*

Interval History: *The patient continues to have severe abdominal pain and severe vaginal bleeding.*

Physical Examination: *The cervix is closed and unfavorable.*

Labs:
- *CBC 5.0> 9.1/28.5< 60,000*
- *Fibrinogen: 100 mg/dL (high)*
- *US: Large amounts of blood between the placenta and uterus*
- *Blood type: O-*

Fetal Heart Monitor:
- *Nonreassuring with the presence of beat-to-beat variability*
- *Late decelerations present*

What is the major complication of placental abruption that this patient is experiencing?

a. Anemia

b. ABO incompatibility

c. Disseminated intravascular coagulation (DIC)

d. Thrombocytopenia

Answer c. Disseminated intravascular coagulation (DIC)

DIC and fetal loss are the most dangerous complications of placental abruption. DIC is managed by transfusion of blood products to stabilize the patient. ABO incompatibility itself is not a complication of abruption. All Rh-negative patients should be given RhoGAM to prevent Rh isoimmunization. This will prevent complications in the next pregnancy.

What is the next step in the management of this patient?

a. Delivery of the fetus via C-section

b. Delivery of the fetus vaginally

c. Transfusion of 2 units of packed red blood cells

d. Transfusion of 2 units of platelets

Answer a. Delivery of the fetus via C-section

The fetal heart monitor is showing a nonreassuring heart rate with late decelerations. Late decelerations show that the baby is not getting enough oxygenated blood from the placenta. Late decelerations means the baby has to be delivered urgently. The transfusions of both platelets and PRBCs can be done during the C-section. Nothing should delay the C-section.

Interval History: *The patient underwent emergency C-section and gave birth to a baby boy. She was immediately transferred to the intensive care unit for DIC management.*

CHAPTER 4

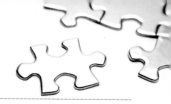

THIRD TRIMESTER COMPLICATIONS

CASE 1: Preeclampsia

CC: *"I'm pregnant and have a headache."*

Setting: *Outpatient*

VS: *BP, 150/90 mm Hg; P, 90 beats/min; R, beats/min; R, 16 breaths/min; T, 98.3°F*

HPI: *A 29-year-old G_1P_0 with an intrauterine pregnancy (IUP) at 37 weeks' gestation presents to the office for a routine prenatal visit. The patient states that she has a headache since this morning. She has no past medical history, no past surgical history, is taking no medications, and has no allergies. She denies visual disturbance, epigastric pain, nausea, and vomiting.*

ROS:
- *Fetal movement: Present*
- *Contractions: Absent*
- *Leakage of fluid: Absent*
- *Vaginal bleeding: Absent*

What is the next step in the management of this patient?

a. Betamethasone
b. Labetalol
c. Magnesium sulfate

d. Nonstress test
e. Urinalysis (UA)

Answer e. Urinalysis (UA)

This patient may be experiencing symptoms of preeclampsia. Preeclampsia is defined as an elevation in blood pressure (BP) and proteinuria that develops after 20 weeks' gestation. The patient should have a UA to measure the amount of protein in the urine. Administering any medication at this point would be premature; the patient needs a diagnosis before starting any treatment. A nonstress test may be done to monitor the baby, but this should be done after the UA.

On the CCS, the initial order set should include a complete blood count (CBC), comprehensive metabolic panel (CMP), UA, 24-hour urine protein, maternal monitoring, and fetal monitoring.

If preeclampsia is being considered, transfer the patient to the inpatient floor!

Which of the following organs is most affected by preeclampsia?

a. Brain

b. Heart

c. Kidneys

d. Liver

e. Spleen

Answer c. Kidneys

Preeclampsia causes endothelial damage. The kidneys are most susceptible to this damage. The first sign that the kidneys are being damaged is proteinuria. The myocardium is not directly affected by preeclampsia.

Move the clock forward to the next available test result.

Setting: *Inpatient unit (labor and delivery)*

Interval History: *The patient continues to have a headache. She denies visual disturbances.*

Maternal VS: *BP, 156/96 mm Hg; P, 89 beats/min*

Fetal Monitoring: *Accelerations are present, good variability, no decelerations*

Labs:
- *CBC: White blood cells (WBCs), $6.3 \times 10^3/\mu L$; hemoglobin (Hgb), 11.3 g/dL; hematocrit (Hct), 33.9%; platelets: $300 \times 10^3/\mu L$*
- *CMP: Sodium, 127 mmol/L; potassium, 4.7 mmol/L; chloride, 100 mmol/L; bicarbonate, 26 mmol/L; blood urea nitrogen (BUN), 10 mg/dL; creatinine, 0.9 mg/dL; glucose, 110 mg/dL*
- *ALT: 22 IU/L AST: 20 IU/L*
- *UA: 2+ protein*

What is the next step in the management of this patient?

a. Phenytoin

b. Magnesium sulfate

c. Delivery via C-section

d. Induction of labor

Answer b. Magnesium sulfate

Patients with preeclampsia should undergo seizure prophylaxis with magnesium sulfate after they are diagnosed. Preeclampsia is classified as either mild or severe.

	Mild	Severe
Hypertension (BP, mm Hg)	>140/90	>160/110
Proteinuria	1+-2+	3+
Edema	Peripheral areas	Generalized
Mental status changes	No	Yes
Vision change	No	Yes
Change in liver function tests	No	Yes

Eclampsia is the occurrence of tonic clonic seizure in a patient with preeclampsia.

The only definitive treatment for preeclampsia and eclampsia is DELIVERY!

What is the first sign of toxicity with magnesium sulfate?

a. Cardiac arrest
b. Depressed respiratory drive
c. Diminished deep tendon reflexes
d. Nausea
e. Headache

Answer c. Diminished deep tendon reflexes.

Magnesium sulfate is a peripheral vasodilator that, when infused quickly, may cause a drop in BP. Some symptoms of this drop in BP are nausea and headache. These are not signs of toxicity. Although toxicity is rare in women who have normal kidney function, it should still be monitored for in every patient. The first sign of toxicity is diminished deep tendon reflexes. As the toxicity progresses, respiratory drive decreases and may progress to cardiac arrest.

Move the clock forward 1 hour.

Interval History: *The patient continues to have a headache.*

Cervical Exam: *The cervix is closed, not effaced, and is at station-3.*

What is the next step in the management of this patient?

a. Administration of betamethasone
b. C-section now
c. Induction of labor with oxytocin
d. Induction of labor with misoprostol

Answer d. Induction of labor with misoprostol

Patients with mild preeclampsia can undergo induction and vaginal delivery as long as the fetus and mother are stable. Betamethasone is only given to patients who are preterm. Betamethasone helps mature the fetal lung to decrease newborn respiratory distress. Induction of labor with an "unfavorable" cervix, as in this patient, should be done with misoprostol. Oxytocin will help augment contractions after the cervix is open.

Patients with severe preeclampsia should receive BP control with hydralazine.

Where is oxytocin produced?

a. Hypothalamus

b. Posterior pituitary

c. Anterior pituitary

d. Uterus

e. Ovary

Latent phase
unfavorable
cervix → miso
prostol

Active phase
unfavorable cervix - oxy
(protracted cervix tocin)

Answer a. Hypothalamus

Oxytocin in produced in the hypothalamus and stored in the posterior pituitary. It is released from the posterior pituitary based on stimulation of the uterus by contractions. It is a polypeptide hormone (Figure 4-1).

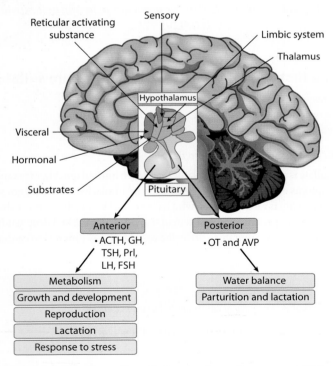

Figure 4-1. Hypothalamic neuropeptides and pituitary release of hormones. ACTH, adrenocorticotropic hormone; AVP, argininevasopressin; FSH, follicle-stimulating hormone; GH, growth hormone; LH, luteinizing hormone; OT, oxytocin; Prl, prolactin; TSH, thyroid-stimulating hormone. (Reproduced with permission from Molina PE. *Endocrine Physiology,* 4th ed. New York: McGraw-Hill; 2013.)

Oxytocin contracts breast myoepithelial cells; therefore, breast milk will not be released for a few days (Figure 4-2).

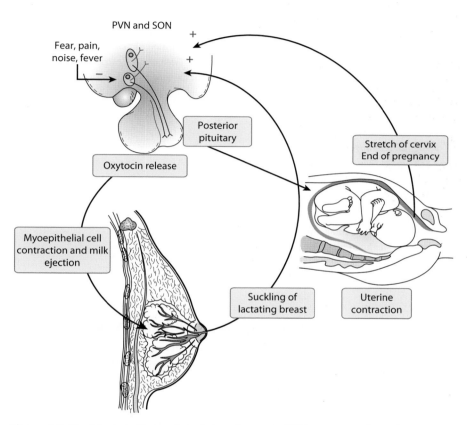

Figure 4-2. Physiological effects and regulation of oxytocin. PVN, paraventricular nucleus; SON, supraoptic nucleus. (Reproduced with permission from Molina PE. *Endocrine Physiology*, 4th ed. New York: McGraw-Hill; 2013.)

Interval History: *The patient continues to receive magnesium sulfate and delivers a healthy baby girl. The patient remains on magnesium sulfate for 24 hours after delivery.*

CASE 2: Premature Rupture of Membranes

CC: *"I felt a gush of fluid."*

Setting: *Emergency department*

VS: *BP, 110/80 mm Hg; P, 88 beats/min; R, 12 breaths/min; T, 98.6°F*

HPI: *A 29-year-old G_3P_{1011} with an IUP at 37 weeks' gestation presents to the emergency department because of a gush of fluid from her vagina. The patient denies any other complaints. States that she was watching TV when she felt the gush. The fluid appeared clear.*

ROS:
- *Fetal movement: Present*
- *Contractions: Absent*
- *Vaginal bleeding: Absent*
- *Leakage of fluid: Present*

PE:
- *CVS: Normal*
- *Lungs: Normal*
- *Abd: gravid, nontender, nondistended, +BS*
- *Ext: No edema bilaterally*

What is the next step in the management of this patient?

a. Administer betamethasone

b. Digital cervical examination

c. Fetal fibronectin

d. Sterile speculum examination

Answer d. Sterile speculum examination

During the speculum examination, pooling may be seen. Pooling is a collection of amniotic fluid located in the posterior fornix. A sample of this fluid should be taken for a nitrazine test and for a ferning test. Nitrazine paper will turn blue in the presence of amniotic fluid. Blue means the fluid is basic or alkaline. The ferning test is done by placing some of the fluid on a slide and examining it under the microscope. If the fluid is amniotic fluid, then a fernlike pattern will form on the slide (Figure 4-3).

Fetal fibronectin is a test that will help determine if a woman is in preterm labor. It should be done on patients that present with contractions before the 35th week of gestation. Fetal fibronectin is a glycoprotein that acts like the glue that holds the uterus and the placenta together. This test should be done on women who have *intact* fetal membranes, abdominal contractions, and cervical dilation *less than* 3 cm and who have not had sexual relations in the past 48 hours.

Betamethasone is not administered before a diagnosis of premature labor is made. There is no point in giving betamethasone to increase fetal lung surfactant production unless you are planning to deliver the baby.

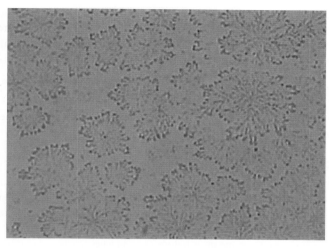

Figure 4-3. Ferning pattern that develops when amniotic fluid is dried. (Reproduced with permission from Tintinalli JE, Stapczynski J, Ma OJ, et al. *Tintinalli's Emergency Medicine: A Comprehensive Study Guide,* 7th ed. New York: McGraw-Hill; 2011.)

Steroids increase surfactant production from type 2 pneumocytes.
• Lung volume increases.
• Lung compliance increases.

Move the clock ahead to the next interaction.

Interval History: *A sterile speculum exam was done. Pooling was seen and the fluid turned the nitrazine paper blue. The cervix appeared closed.*
   Nitrazine paper
   Blue = Basic = pH 7 = Amniotic fluid
   Yellow = Acid = pH 4 = Vaginal fluid

What is the diagnosis?

a. Premature rupture of membranes
b. Prolonged rupture of membranes

c. Preterm premature rupture of membranes
d. Active labor

Answer a. Premature rupture of membranes

Premature rupture of membranes is defined as rupture of the membranes before active labor or contractions begin. Prolonged rupture of membranes occurs when the membranes have been ruptured for more than 24 hours without delivery of the fetus. Preterm premature rupture of membranes occurs when there is rupture of the membranes before

37 weeks' gestation and the patient is not in active labor. Active labor includes that the patient has contractions and cervical dilation. After the diagnosis of premature rupture of membranes is made, you should limit the number of digital examinations. Digital examinations introduce bacteria and increase the risk of infection and chorioamnionitis.

What is the next step in management of this patient?

a. Betamethasone

b. Magnesium sulfate

c. Tocolytic such as terbutaline

d. Induction of labor with oxytocin

Answer d. Induction of labor with oxytocin

This patient is at term at 37 weeks of gestation. There is no reason to mature the fetus' lungs with betamethasone, stop labor with tocolytics, or administer magnesium sulfate for seizure prophylaxis or as a tocolytic. This patient should undergo induction of labor with oxytocin.

If the patient was preterm, meaning before 24 to 34 weeks, then betamethasone should be given to mature the fetal lungs. In patients with preterm premature rupture of membranes, antibiotics should also be administered. The antibiotics of choice are ampicillin and azithromycin.

What is the biggest complication of premature rupture of membranes?

a. Chorioamnionitis

b. Preterm labor

c. Vasa previa

d. Placenta abruption

e. Placenta previa

Answer a. Chorioamnionitis

Chorioamnionitis is an infection of the amniotic fluid, membranes, or placenta. This is not only a cause of premature rupture of membranes but also a complication. Patients with prolonged or premature rupture of membranes may develop an infection secondary to excessive digital examinations. Patients often develop leukocytosis, fever, uterine tenderness, and tachycardia. If chorioamnionitis develops, the fetus is at increased risk for infection and neonatal sepsis.

Premature rupture of membranes is associated with preterm labor and placental abruption. However, the most feared complication is chorioamnionitis.

If at any time chorioamnionitis is diagnosed, the patient needs to be delivered and intravenous ampicillin and gentamicin started. Alternatives are ampicillin–sulbactam or ticarcillin–clavulanic acid.

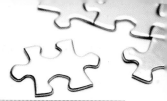

CHAPTER 5

Rh INCOMPATIBILITY

CASE 1: Rh Incompatibility

CC: *"I'm pregnant and have type O negative blood."*

Setting: *Outpatient*

VS: *BP, 115/75 mm Hg; P, 82 beats/min; R, 12 breaths/min; T, 98.6°F*

HPI: *A 29-year-old G_2P_{1001} with an intrauterine pregnancy (IUP) at 8 weeks' gestation presents to the office for a routine prenatal examination. The patient states that with her first pregnancy, she was told that she had blood type O negative. She states that she read online that this could be a problem with the second pregnancy, and she is extremely concerned.*

ROS:
- *Contractions: Absent*
- *Vaginal bleeding: Absent*
- *Leakage of fluid: Absent*

PE:
- *CVS: Normal*
- *Lungs: Normal*
- *Abd: Nontender, nondistended, +BS*
- *Ext: No edema*

What is the next step in the management of this patient?

a. Indirect Coombs titer

b. CBC

c. Blood type

d. Kleihauer-Betke smear

e. Percutaneous umbilical blood sample (PUBS)

Answer a. Indirect Coombs titer

This patient already stated that she has blood type O negative and was pregnant once before. Indirect Coombs titers will show if the patient is "sensitized," meaning her body made antibodies to the fetal blood, or "unsensitized," meaning her body did not make antibodies to the fetal blood (Figure 5-1).

A Kleihauer-Betke smear is used to detect fetal—maternal hemorrhage. It is a sample of maternal blood used to measure the amount of fetal blood mixing with maternal blood.

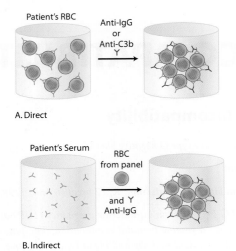

Figure 5-1. Coombs test. RBC, red blood cell. (Used with permission from Dr. Peter Marks in Bunn HF. *Pathophysiology of Blood Disorders*. New York: McGraw-Hill; 2011.)

Maternal blood is exposed to acid. Hemoglobin A denatures, and the cells look like "ghosts." The fetal cells are left intact because hemoglobin F is resistant to acid.

PUBS is a procedure done on the infant to determine the fetal hematocrit and reticulocyte count, but it is premature at this point (Figure 5-2). PUBS also tests for antibodies in fetal serum. Rh isoimmunization is a problem with antibodies in maternal serum. PUBS also leads to fetal loss in 1% to 2% of those sampled. PUBS would be done after the status of Rh incompatibility is determined and the bilirubin level found in the amniotic fluid is found to be high.

Rh incompatibility occurs when the mother is Rh *negative* and the baby is Rh *positive*. It is not a problem in the first pregnancy because the mother has not yet developed antibodies to the fetal blood. During the first pregnancy, fetal red blood cells (RBCs) may pass through the placenta and into the mother's bloodstream. This will allow her body to make the antibodies. This often happens at delivery but may occur any time there is a hemorrhage, including during spontaneous abortions. When the mother starts to make antibodies to the Rh-positive blood, the second Rh-positive baby will be attacked by the antibodies.

Kleihauer Betke test:
- Detects fetal blood in maternal blood
- HgA denatures with acid
- HgF stable with acid

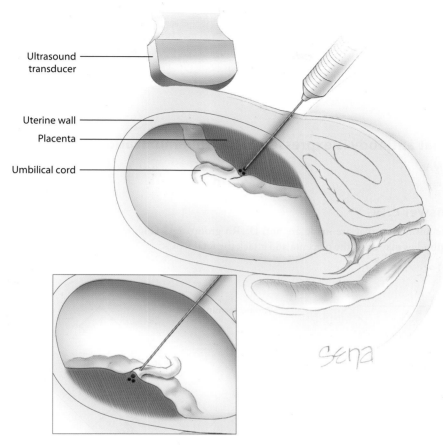

Ultrasound transducer

Uterine wall

Placenta

Umbilical cord

Figure 5-2. Percutaneous umbilical blood sampling. (Reproduced with permission from Cunningham F, Leveno K, Bloom S, et al. *Williams Obstetrics,* 23rd ed. New York: McGraw-Hill; 2010.)

Scenarios in which maternal and fetal blood may mix:
• Amniocentesis (any invasive prenatal testing)
• Abortions (spontaneous and induced)
• Vaginal bleeding
• Placental abruption
• Delivery
• Trauma

On the CCS, the following should be in the initial order set: a complete blood count (CBC), comprehensive metabolic panel (CMP), indirect Coombs test, blood type and screen, rapid plasma reagin (RPR), HIV, gonorrhea, Chlamydia, Pap smear, and rubella. Do not forget that this is her initial prenatal visit, so all of the proper testing should be done, not only the indirect Coombs test.

What antibody is expressed in Rh isoimmunization?

a. IgA

b. IgE

c. IgG

d. IgM

Answer c. IgG

The antibodies that are made are anti-D (Rh group) IgG (Figures 5-3 and 5-4). These antibodies may cross the placenta and attack the fetal RBCs.

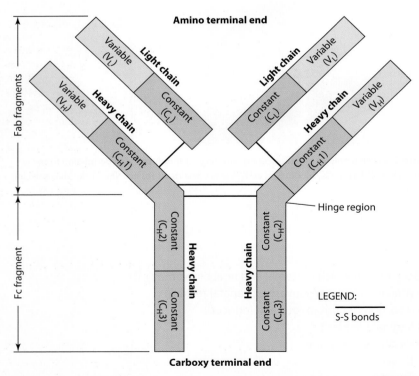

Figure 5-3. IgG configuration. (Reproduced with permission from Brooks GF, Carrol KC, Butel J, Morse S. *Jawetz, Melnick, & Adelberg's Medical Microbiology*, 25th ed. New York: McGraw-Hill, 2010.)

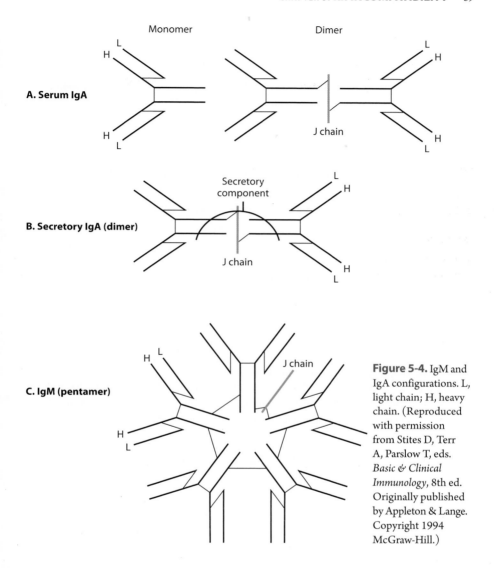

Monomer   Dimer

A. Serum IgA

J chain

B. Secretory IgA (dimer)

Secretory
component

J chain

C. IgM (pentamer)

J chain

Figure 5-4. IgM and IgA configurations. L, light chain; H, heavy chain. (Reproduced with permission from Stites D, Terr A, Parslow T, eds. *Basic & Clinical Immunology*, 8th ed. Originally published by Appleton & Lange. Copyright 1994 McGraw-Hill.)

What ethnicity has the highest rate of Rh-negative mothers?

a. Asians
b. African Americans

c. Whites
d. Hispanics

Answer c. Whites

A total of 15% of whites, 8% of African Americans, 7% of Hispanics, and less than 1% of Asians are Rh negative. The greater the rate of Rh negativity, the greater the rate of Rh isoimmunization. A person cannot develop anti-Rh (D) antibodies if the blood is Rh positive. Also, if the father is Rh negative and the mother is Rh negative, they cannot have an Rh-positive child.

Move the clock forward to the next prenatal visit (4 weeks).

Setting: *Outpatient clinic*

Interval History: *The patient is now at 16 weeks' gestation. She denies any contractions, vaginal bleeding, and leakage of fluid. She also denies fetal movement.*

Labs:
- *The patient's routine prenatal laboratory test results return within normal limits.*
- *Indirect Coombs antibody titer: 1:16*

What is the next step in the management of this patient?

a. Administer anti-D immunoglobulin (RhoGAM) now

b. Amniocentesis

c. PUBS

d. Maternal bilirubin level

Answer b. Amniocentesis

An amniocentesis should be done between 16 and 20 weeks' gestation to evaluate the fetal blood type. The mother has a significant antibody titer to anti-D IgG. The mother is considered "sensitized" when the titer is 1:4. However, the patient can be managed as one with a normal pregnancy until the titer rises to 1:16 or more. If this happens, the fetal blood type needs to be checked. Maternal bilirubin levels will not increase in hemolytic disease of the newborn. PUBS is still premature at this point. PUBS would be done if the bilirubin level on amniocentesis was found to be high. A high bilirubin level in the amniotic fluid means the baby is probably anemic. If it is thought that the baby is anemic, then a PUBS should be done.

After a mother is "sensitized," RhoGAM will not work.

Move the clock ahead 1 week.

Interval History: *The patient is feeling well and presents at 20 weeks' gestation for the results of her amniocentesis done last week.*

Amniocentesis:
- *Fetal blood cells are O+.*
- *Fetal bilirubin is low.*

What is the next step in the management of this patient?

a. Repeat amniocentesis in 1 to 2 weeks

b. Repeat amniocentesis in 2 to 3 weeks

c. PUBS

d. Fetal blood transfusion

Answer b. Repeat amniocentesis in 2 to 3 weeks

As long as the fetal bilirubin level remains low, an amniocentesis should be done every 2 to 3 weeks to monitor the level. As the level rises, an amniocentesis should be done more often. If the level is considered medium, the amniocentesis should be done every 1 to 2 weeks. If the bilirubin level is high, it means that there is a lot of RBC breakdown, and the fetus is probably anemic. When the bilirubin level reaches a high level, a PUBS should be done to monitor the fetal hematocrit. If the fetal hematocrit is low, an intrauterine transfusion may be done.

Hemolytic disease of the newborn results in fetal anemia and extramedullary production of RBCs. Extramedullary production means that the RBCs are produced outside the bone marrow.

> Indirect bilirubin is released from RBC breakdown (Figures 5-5 and 5-6). Bilirubin is neurotoxic in babies

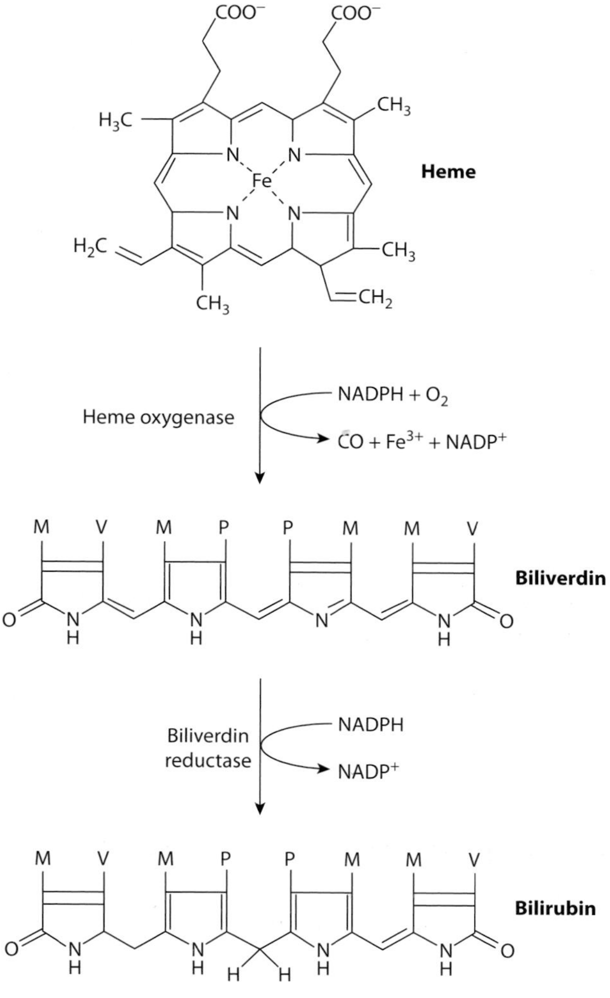

Figure 5-5. Degradation of hemoglobin to bilirubin. (Reproduced with permission from Barrett KE, Barman SM, Boitano S. *Ganong's Review of Medical Physiology*, 24th ed. New York: McGraw-Hill; 2012.)

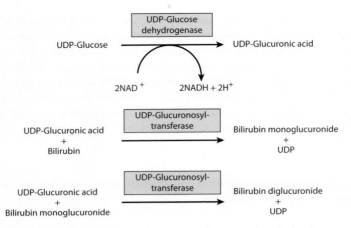

Figure 5-6. Conjugation of bilirubin with glucuronic acid. UDP, uridine diphosphate glucuronyltransferase. (Reproduced with permission from Murray RK, Bender DA, Botham KM, et al. *Harper's Illustrated Biochemistry,* 29th ed. New York: McGraw-Hill; 2012.)

> *Move the clock ahead 2 weeks.*
> *The amniocentesis will be repeated every 2 to 3 weeks to monitor the bilirubin levels in the amniotic fluid. As long as they remain low, no further intervention is needed. If they return to being high, it means the fetus may be anemic, and a PUBS should be done. If the fetus is anemic, then a blood transfusion through PUBS is indicated.*

When should RhoGAM be administered?

a. At 12 weeks' gestation   **c.** At delivery only
b. At 28 weeks' gestation

Answer b. At 28 weeks' gestation

RhoGAM is an anti-D Rh immunoglobulin that is administered routinely at 28 weeks' gestation to Rh-negative mothers. After the baby is delivered, if the baby had Rh-positive blood, RhoGAM should be administered again.

The goal of RhoGAM is to prevent the mother from making antibodies to the fetal blood. It should be administered any time the fetal and maternal blood may mix.

Anytime maternal and fetal blood may mix = Give RhoGAM

RhoGAM should be administered:
• In spontaneous abortions
• At 28 weeks' gestation
• At delivery
• In induced abortions
• During amniocentesis

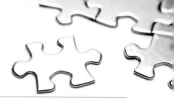

CHAPTER 6

ECTOPIC PREGNANCY

CASE 1: Ectopic Pregnancy

CC: *"I have right lower quadrant abdominal pain."*

Setting: *Emergency department*

VS: *BP, 115/75 mm Hg; P, 82 beats/min; R, 12 breaths/min; T, 98.6°F*

HPI: *An 18-year-old woman presents to the emergency department for right lower quadrant abdominal pain. The pain started suddenly with a sharp, stabbing pain. The patient denies nausea, vomiting, diarrhea, and constipation. Her last menstrual period (LMP) was 6 weeks ago.*

PE:
- *Gen: Awake, alert, oriented ×3, mild pain distress*
- *CVS: Normal*
- *Lungs: Clear bilaterally*
- *Abd: Tender in right lower quadrant (RLQ), rebound tenderness present, nondistended, bowel sounds present*

Which of the following is the next best step in the management of this patient?

a. Complete blood count (CBC)

b. Computed tomography (CT) scan

c. Urine beta-human chorionic gonadotropin (BHCG)

d. Ultrasound

e. Abdominal radiography

Answer c. Urine beta-human chorionic gonadotropin (BHCG)

This patient is presenting with symptoms of RLQ abdominal pain. This could be appendicitis, ovarian cyst, salpingitis, pelvic inflammatory disease, or ectopic pregnancy. The clue to the diagnosis is that the patient's LMP was 6 weeks ago. If the question wants to lead you in a certain direction, it will give you a hint. Urine BHCG should be done on all women of childbearing age with lower abdominal pain. This is done before a CT scan to rule out appendicitis. CBC will not give you a diagnosis. The presence of lower abdominal pain is more important than the menstrual history. Menstrual histories are often inaccurate.

On the CCS, initial orders should include CBC, basic metabolic panel (BMP), urine BHCG, normal saline, nothing by mouth (NPO), and intravenous (IV) morphine.

Move the clock forward to the next available test result.

Interval History: *Patient is feeling better with the morphine.*

Labs:
- CBC: White blood cell count (WBC), 5.1 × 10³/μL; hemoglobin (Hg), 10.3 g/dL; hematocrit (Hct), 30.9%; platelets: 200 × 10³/μL
- BMP: Sodium, 125 mmol/L; potassium, 4.1 mmol/L; blood urea nitrogen (BUN), 10 mg/dL; creatinine, 0.9 mg/dL; glucose, 120 mg/dL
- Urine BHCG: Positive

Which of the following is the strongest risk factor for ectopic pregnancy?

a. Age

b. Use of an intrauterine device

c. Pelvic inflammatory disease

d. Previous ectopic pregnancy

e. Smoking

Answer d. Previous ectopic pregnancy

All of the choices are risk factors for ectopic pregnancy. However, the strongest risk factor is previous ectopic pregnancy.

Risk factors for ectopic pregnancy:
- Previous ectopic pregnancy
- Fallopian tube surgery
- Pelvic inflammatory disease
- Intrauterine devices
- Infertility
- In vitro fertilization
- Multiple sexual partners
- Smoking

Infection scars the fallopian tubes.
Scars in the tubes make eggs implant at wrong place (Figure 6-1).

What is the next step in the management of this patient?

a. Administer methotrexate

b. Laparoscopy

c. Transvaginal ultrasonography

d. Transfusion of packed red blood cells (PRBCs)

Answer c. Transvaginal ultrasonography

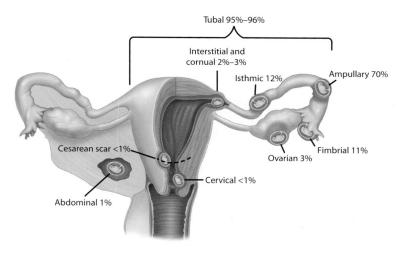

Figure 6-1. Ectopic pregnancy locations. (Reproduced with permission from Cunningham F, Leveno K, Bloom S, et al. *Williams Obstetrics*, 23rd ed. New York: McGraw-Hill; 2010.)

Just because the patient has right lower quadrant pain and is pregnant does not mean this is definitely an ectopic pregnancy. The ectopic pregnancy should be localized first with ultrasonography (Figure 6-2). Administering methotrexate or doing a laparoscopy would not be done before confirming the location of the pregnancy with ultrasonography. The diagnosis of ectopic needs to be made. The patient may have an intrauterine pregnancy.

Move the clock forward to the next available test result.

Interval History: *Transvaginal ultrasonography shows a fetal pole in the right fallopian tube measuring 3 cm.*
    On the CCS, when the diagnosis of ectopic pregnancy is made, transfer the patient to the inpatient unit.

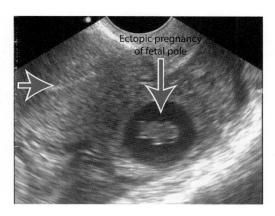

Figure 6-2. Ectopic pregnancy on transvaginal ultrasonography. (Reproduced with permission from Ma OJ, Mateer JR, Blaivas M. *Emergency Ultrasound*, 2nd ed. New York: McGraw-Hill; 2008).

What is the next step in the management of this patient?

a. Administer methotrexate
b. Emergent salpingectomy

c. Transfuse 2 units of packed red blood cells (RBCs)
d. Laparoscopy

Answer a. Administer methotrexate

Methotrexate is the medical treatment for an ectopic pregnancy. It may be administered to patients after baseline labs are drawn. These baseline laboratory studies should include CBC, CMP (including liver function tests), and BHCG. Emergency salpingectomy is not indicated at this time. Salpingectomy would be considered if methotrexate did not work or there was tubal rupture. If the ectopic pregnancy had ruptured, an emergency surgery or transfusion may have been needed.

98% of ectopic pregnancies occur in a fallopian tube (Figure 6-3).

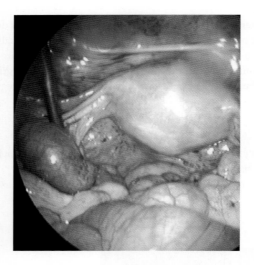

Figure 6-3. Laparoscopic view of an ectopic pregnancy. (Used with permission from Doody D. In Hoffman BL, Schorge J, Halvorson L, et al (eds). *Williams Gynecology,* 2nd ed. New York: McGraw-Hill; 2012).

Salpingostomy = Opening of the fallopian tube (Figure 6-4)
Salpingectomy = Removal of the fallopian tube

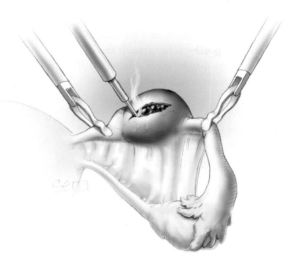

Figure 6-4. Salpingostomy. (Reproduced with permission from Hoffman BL, Schorge J, Halvorson L, et al (eds). *Williams Gynecology,* 2nd ed. New York: McGraw-Hill; 2012).

Contraindications to methotrexate use:
- Immunodeficiency
- Noncompliant patients
- Hepatotoxicity
- Ectopic pregnancy >3.5 cm
- Fetal heartbeat

Move the clock forward 1 week.

Interval History: *Methotrexate was given, and BHCG was drawn 1 week later. BHCG dropped 20% since the last BHCG.*

What is the next step in the management of this patient?

a. Administer a second dose of methotrexate.

b. Refer for salpingostomy.

c. Repeat BHCG in 1 week.

d. Follow up when the patient becomes pregnant again.

Answer c. Repeat BHCG in 1 week.

Methotrexate should decrease the BHCG by 15% in 1 week. If this occurs, then there was an optimal reaction to the methotrexate, and the patient should continue to have BHCG checked every week until the level reaches zero. If the BHCG did not decrease 15%, then a second dose of methotrexate may be given. On repeat BHCG, if there still is not a 15% decrease, then surgical intervention will be required.

Methotrexate is a folate antagonist.
Long-term use leads to liver and lung fibrosis.
Single-dose therapy has no major adverse effects.

Efficacy of methotrexate = Efficacy of surgery

Interval History: *After administration of methotrexate, the BHCG level was followed every week until it reached zero.*

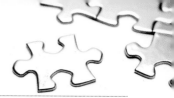

CHAPTER 7

LABOR AND DELIVERY

CASE 1: Labor and Delivery

CC: *"I think I'm in labor."*

Setting: *Inpatient unit (labor and delivery)*

VS: *BP, 115/75 mm Hg; P, 82 beats/min; R, 12 breaths/min; T, 98.6°F*

HPI: *A 25-year-old G_1P_0 with an intrauterine pregnancy (IUP) at 38 weeks' gestation presents to the labor and delivery unit stating that she thinks she is in labor. She has had routine prenatal care. She states that she has generalized abdominal pain that comes and goes. The pain has been going on for about 5 hours and is starting to become regular. She thinks it is contractions.*

ROS:
- *Contractions: Present*
- *Fetal movement: Present*
- *Vaginal bleeding: Absent*
- *Leakage of fluid: Absent*

PE:
- *Gen: Awake, alert, oriented ×3, mild pain distress*
- *CVS: S_1S_2 + RRR no m/r/g*
- *Lungs: CTA bilaterally*
- *Abd: Gravid*
- *Ext: 1+ edema bilaterally*

What is the next step in the management of this patient?

a. Digital cervical examination   **c.** Transabdominal US

b. Transvaginal ultrasonography (US)   **d.** Nonstress test

Answer a. Digital cervical examination

Physical examination is imperative in all patients and is completed before any testing should be done. Physical examination with a digital cervical examination determines if the patient is in labor. There are several stages to labor, and the digital cervical examination will identify which stage she is in. Transvaginal US is not done when a patient is in active labor. Transabdominal US may be done at the bedside to assure that the fetus is in a cephalic presentation (head down) and not breech.

There are three stages of labor. Stage one is split into active and latent phases. The latent phase is from the onset of labor to 4 cm of dilation. There is variation in the amount of time it takes to go through the stages, depending on if it is the patient's first baby (primipara) or has had a baby before (multipara).

> Primipara = First baby
> Multipara = More than one baby

On the CCS, the following should be included in the initial order set: complete blood count (CBC), complete metabolic panel (CMP), digital cervical examination, abdominal US, intravenous fluids (IVF), and fetal electronic monitoring.

> *Move the clock forward 1 hour.*
>
> **Interval History:** *The patient states that her abdominal pain is worsening.*
>
> **Cervical Examination:** *2 cm, 50% effaced, and -2 station*
>
> **Bedside Abdominal US:** *Fetal in cephalic presentation (head down)*

What stage of labor is this patient in?

a. Latent phase

b. Active phase

c. Stage 2

d. Stage 3

Answer a. Latent phase

Stage 1 is divided into two substages, the latent and active phases. The latent phase starts with the onset of regular contractions and ends when the patient is 4 cm dilated. This may take up to 7 hours in a primipara and 5 hours in a multipara (Figure 7-1). Active labor starts at 4 cm of dilation and ends when the patient is fully dilated. Primipara patients should

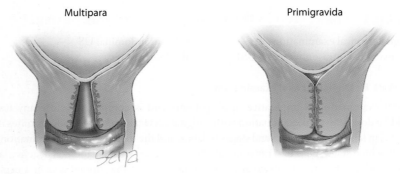

Multipara   Primigravida

Figure 7-1. Cervical dilation and effacement before labor. (Reproduced with permission from Cunningham F, Leveno K, Bloom S, et al. *Williams Obstetrics,* 23rd ed. New York: McGraw-Hill; 2010.)

dilate 1 cm per hour during this phase. In multipara patients, 1.2 cm per hour of dilation is normal.

During stage 1, the maternal blood pressure and pulse, fetal heart rate, and uterine contractions need to be monitored. The cervix should be checked with a digital cervical examination every 2 hours to monitor progression

> Dilation = How many centimeters the cervix is open (Figure 7-2)
> Effacement = How soft the cervix is (Figure 7-3)
> Station = How high the baby's head is in relation to the pelvic bones (Figure 7-4)

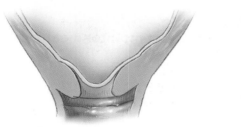 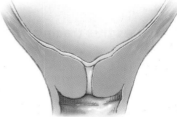

Figure 7-2. Effacement (thinning of the cervix). (Reproduced with permission from Cunningham F, Leveno K, Bloom S, et al. *Williams Obstetrics,* 23rd ed. New York: McGraw-Hill; 2010.)

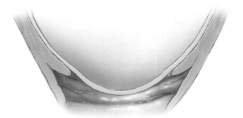 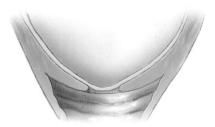

Figure 7-3. Complete effacement in multipara vs primipara. In a primipara, the dilation is minimal, but in a multipara, dilation is also occurring. (Reproduced with permission from Cunningham F, Leveno K, Bloom S, et al. *Williams Obstetrics,* 23rd ed. New York: McGraw-Hill; 2010.)

Move the clock forward 1 hour.

Interval History: *The nurse calls because there is an abnormality on the fetal heart monitor.*

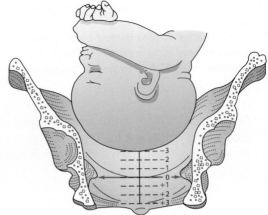

Figure 7-4. Fetal station. (Reproduced with permission from Benson RC. *Handbook of Obstetrics & Gynecology,* 8th ed. New York: Lange and McGraw-Hill; 1983.)

What does this tracing on the fetal heart monitor mean?

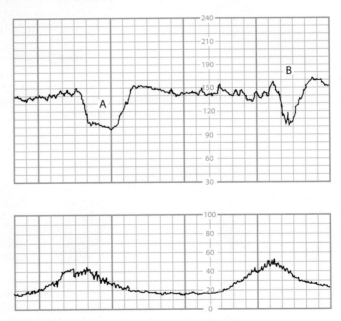

Figure 7-5. Variable decelerations. A and B are the decelerations. (Adapted with permission from Künzel W. *Fetal Heart Rate Monitoring: Clinical Practice and Pathophysiology.* Berlin, Springer-Verlag; 1985, as in Cunningham F, Leveno K, Bloom S, et al. *Williams Obstetrics,* 23rd ed. New York: McGraw-Hill; 2010.)

a. The baby is hypoxic.
b. The baby's head is being compressed.

c. The umbilical cord is compressed.

Answer c. The umbilical cord is compressed.

Variable decelerations are a decrease in heart rate with a return to the base line that has *no* relationship with the contractions. The umbilical vein is more sensitive to compression than the umbilical artery. This alters fetal heart rate by impeding preload and afterload.

Electronic Fetal Monitoring: *The top line is the fetal heart rate while the bottom is maternal contractions.*

The fetal heart rate is normally 110 to 160 beats/min

Tachycardia >160 beats/min, Bradycardia <110 beats/min

Accelerations are increases in the fetal heart rate by 15 beats/min for 15 to 20 seconds. It should occur twice an hour. This is a good sign and is reassuring.

Variability is the irregular fluctuations of the baseline (Figure 7-6). More variability = Good sign

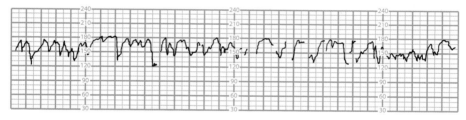

Figure 7-6. Variability. (Adapted with permission from National Institute of Child Health and Human Development Research Planning Workshop. Electronic fetal heart rate monitoring: Research guidelines for integration. *Am J Obstet Gynecol* 1997;177:1385) as in Cunningham F, Leveno K, Bloom S, et al. *Williams Obstetrics,* 23rd ed. New York: McGraw-Hill; 2010.)

If no accelerations have occurred in 1 hour; then the fetus may be sleeping. Stimulate with cervical examination or vibroacoustic stimulation. Decelerations are decreases in the fetal heart rate. They need to be analyzed in relation to the uterine contractions.

Early decelerations: Decreases in heart rate that occurs with contractions. Early decelerations = Fetus' head being compressed (Figure 7-7).

Variable decelerations: Decreases in fetal heart rate *not* occurring with contractions (Figures 7-5 and 7-8). Fetal heart rate returns to baseline. Variable decelerations = Umbilical cord being compressed

Late decelerations: Decreases in fetal heart rate after contraction has started (Figures 7-9). No return in fetal heart rate until contraction has ended. The fetus is hypoxic. This is an indication to do an emergency C-section.

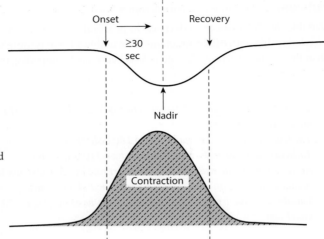

Figure 7-7. Early decelerations. (Reproduced with permission from Cunningham F, Leveno K, Bloom S, et al. *Williams Obstetrics,* 23rd ed. New York: McGraw-Hill; 2010.)

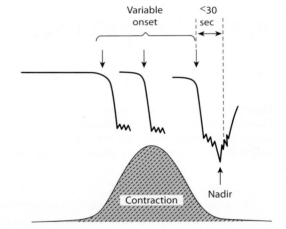

Figure 7-8. Variable decelerations. (Reproduced with permission from Cunningham F, Leveno K, Bloom S, et al. *Williams Obstetrics,* 23rd ed. New York: McGraw-Hill; 2010.)

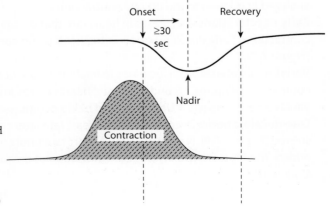

Figure 7-9. Late decelerations. (Reproduced with permission from Cunningham F, Leveno K, Bloom S, et al. *Williams Obstetrics,* 23rd ed. New York: McGraw-Hill; 2010.)

What is the next step in the management of this patient?

a. Emergency C-section

b. Have the patient change position

c. Artificial rupture of membranes

d. Augment labor with oxytocin

Answer b. Have the patient change position

Variable decelerations are associated with compression of the umbilical cord. If the mother changes position to a left lateral position, the pressure may come off the umbilical cord. Augmentation with oxytocin or artificial rupture of membranes will increase the stress on the baby, causing increases in heart rate or decelerations. Augmentation of labor is never indicated as a treatment of decelerations. Decelerations are an indication that the baby is in distress. Augmentation will worsen this distress. Augmentation of labor is indicated when the labor is progressing slowly. C-section is not indicated at this time, but it may be needed if the fetal heart rate does not return to baseline.

> *Move the clock forward by 5 minutes.*
>
> **Interval History:** *The fetal heart rate has returned to normal, and no decelerations are seen.*
>
> **Cervical Examination 2 Hours Later:** *4 cm dilated, 80% effaced, and -2 station*

Which stage of labor is the patient in?

a. Latent

b. Active

c. Stage 2

d. Stage 3

Answer b. Active stage

The active stage of labor starts at 4 cm of dilation. In primiparas, the cervix should dilate 1 cm per hour. In multiparas, the cervix should dilate 1.2 cm every hour.

> • Stage 1
>   • Latent phase = Regular contraction to 4 cm dilated
>   • Active phase = 4 cm to fully dilated
> • Stage 2 = Fully dilated to delivery of the baby
> • Stage 3 = Delivery of the baby until delivery of the placenta

> *Move the clock forward 2 hours.*
>
> **Interval History:** *The patient is feeling stronger contractions*
>
> **Cervical Examination 2 Hours Later:** *5 cm, 80% effaced, and -2 station*
>
> **Fetal Monitoring:** *Reassuring, + acceleration, no decelerations*
> *Uterine contractions appear weaker.*

What is the diagnosis of this patient?

a. Arrest of cervical dilation

b. Malpresentation

c. Protracted cervical dilation

d. Normal labor

Answer c. Protracted cervical dilation

The patient is in active labor, and cervical dilation should occur at 1 cm per hour. It has been 2 hours, and only 1 cm of dilation has occurred. This is protracted cervical dilation, meaning it is taking longer than it is supposed to. Arrest of cervical dilation means the cervix is not dilating at all. Malpresentation means the baby is presenting any way other than with the head down. "Breech birth" is one type of malpresentation. This was already established with ultrasonography at the beginning of the case.

Protracted and arrest of cervical dilation may occur because of the 3Ps:
• Power: Inadequate uterine contractions
• Passenger: Baby is too big or in the wrong position
• Passage: Baby is bigger than the pelvis (cephalopelvic disorder)

Protracted cervical dilation = Less than 1.2 cm in primipara or 1.5 cm in multipara in 1 hour
Arrest of cervical dilation = No dilation of cervix in 1 hour

How do you treat this?

a. Administer magnesium sulfate.

b. Administer oxytocin.

c. Perform a C-section.

d. Give it more time.

Answer b. Administer oxytocin.

It appears that the uterine contractions are weak, so augmentation with oxytocin should be done. If the diagnosis is cephalopelvic disorder, C-section should be done. This means the baby is larger than the birth canal. Magnesium sulfate is administered to patients with preeclampsia.

Move the clock forward 4 hours.

Interval History: *Oxytocin was administered, and the uterine contractions are increasing.*

Cervical Examination 4 Hours Later: *Fully dilated, 100% effaced, -1 station*

Which stage of labor is the patient in?

a. Stage 1, active

b. Stage 1, latent

c. Stage 2

d. Stage 3

Answer c. Stage 2

Stage 2 labor starts with a fully dilated cervix and ends with the delivery of the baby (Figure 7-10). The descent of the fetal head will determine the progression of this stage. Delivery of the fetus includes these cardinal movements.

- Engagement of the head (Figure 7-11)
  - The head enters the pelvis.
- Flexion
- Descent
  - Maternal pushing augments this process.
- Internal rotation (Figure 7-12)
  - The fetal head reaches the ischial spine, and the fetus starts to rotate.

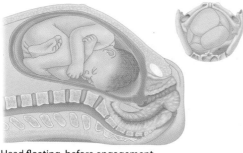
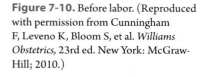

Head floating, before engagement

Figure 7-10. Before labor. (Reproduced with permission from Cunningham F, Leveno K, Bloom S, et al. *Williams Obstetrics,* 23rd ed. New York: McGraw-Hill; 2010.)

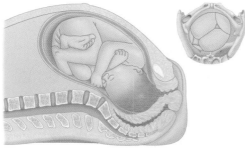

Engagement, descent, flexion

Figure 7-11. Engagement, descent, and flexion. (Reproduced with permission from Cunningham F, Leveno K, Bloom S, et al. *Williams Obstetrics,* 23rd ed. New York: McGraw-Hill; 2010.)

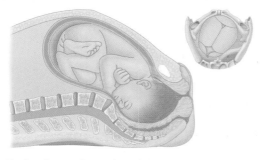

Further descent, internal rotation

Figure 7-12. Descent and internal rotation. (Reproduced with permission from Cunningham F, Leveno K, Bloom S, et al. *Williams Obstetrics,* 23rd ed. New York: McGraw-Hill; 2010.)

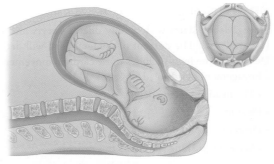

Figure 7-13. Completed rotation; start of extension. (Reproduced with permission from Cunningham F, Leveno K, Bloom S, et al. *Williams Obstetrics,* 23rd ed. New York: McGraw-Hill; 2010.)

Complete rotation, beginning extension

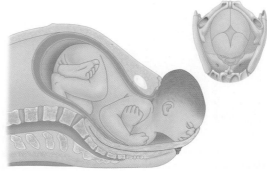

Figure 7-14. Extension. (Reproduced with permission from Cunningham F, Leveno K, Bloom S, et al. *Williams Obstetrics,* 23rd ed. New York: McGraw-Hill; 2010.)

Complete extension

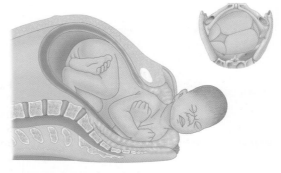

Figure 7-15. External rotation. (Reproduced with permission from Cunningham F, Leveno K, Bloom S, et al. *Williams Obstetrics,* 23rd ed. New York: McGraw-Hill; 2010)

Restitution (external rotation)

- Extension (Figures 7-13 and 7-14)
  - This occurs as the fetal head passes through vagina.
- External rotation (Figure 7-15)
  - External rotation allows the shoulders to pass into the canal.
- Delivery of the anterior shoulder (Figure 7-16)
  - The anterior shoulder goes under the pubic symphysis.
  - Downward pressure should be applied to deliver the anterior shoulder.

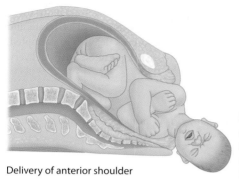

Delivery of anterior shoulder

Figure 7-16. Delivery of the anterior shoulder. (Reproduced with permission from Cunningham F, Leveno K, Bloom S, et al. *Williams Obstetrics,* 23rd ed. New York: McGraw-Hill; 2010.)

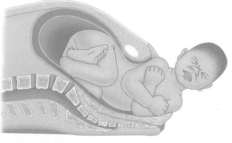

Delivery of posterior shoulder

Figure 7-17. Delivery of the posterior shoulder. (Reproduced with permission from Cunningham F, Leveno K, Bloom S, et al. *Williams Obstetrics,* 23rd ed. New York: McGraw-Hill; 2010.)

- Delivery of the posterior shoulder (Figure 7-17)
  - Upward pressure should be applied to deliver the posterior shoulder.
  - After the posterior shoulder is delivered, the rest of the body will follow

Move the clock forward 2 hours.

Interval History: *The patient has been pushing for 2 hours.*

Cervical Examination: *Fully dilated, 100% effaced, +2 station*

Fetal Heart Monitor: *Reassuring, accelerations are present, good variability, no decelerations*

What is your next step in the management of this patient?

a. C-section

b. Await normal spontaneous vaginal delivery

c. Vacuum-assisted delivery

d. Forceps delivery

Answer b. Await normal spontaneous vaginal delivery

Normal stage 2 labor in a primipara is 30 minutes to 3 hours long. The fetal heart rate is acceptable, and the patient does not have a longer than normal second stage of labor.

C-section, vacuum-assisted delivery, and forceps delivery all have the same indications. These indications include protracted second stage of labor, nonreassuring fetal heart rate, and maternal cardiac or neurologic disease. If vacuum-assisted or forceps delivery is attempted, one must have the availability to immediate C-section if there are complications in the delivery.

Move the clock forward 1 hour.

Interval History: *The patient gave birth to a baby girl via normal spontaneous vaginal delivery. There were no complications.*

What is the next step in the management of this patient?

a. Pull the umbilical cord.
b. Massage the uterus.

c. Inspect for lacerations.

Answer c. Inspect for lacerations.

Inspection is always the first step. After inspection for lacerations, one may monitor for the signs that the placenta is separating from the uterus. These signs include fresh blood per vagina, lengthening of the umbilical cord, the uterine fundus rising, and firmness of the uterus. If these signs are seen, traction may be applied to the umbilical cord to aid in the delivery of the placenta (Figure 7-18). The umbilical cord should never be pulled too hard. Massage of the uterus may be done after the placenta has been removed. This will help the uterus contract and stop the bleeding.

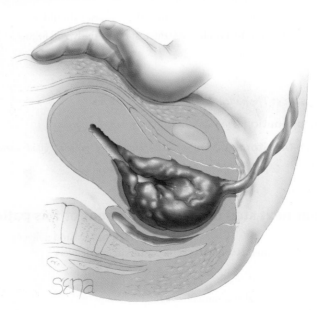

Figure 7-18. Placental delivery. (Reproduced with permission from Cunningham F, Leveno K, Bloom S, et al. *Williams Obstetrics,* 23rd ed. New York: McGraw-Hill; 2010.)

CASE 2: Uterine Rupture

CC: *"I'm in labor, and it hurts."*

Setting: *Inpatient unit (labor and delivery)*

VS: *BP, 115/75 mm Hg; P, 82 beats/min; R, 12 breaths/min; T, 98.6°F*

HPI: *A 31-year-old G_2P_{1001} with an IUP at 39 weeks' gestation present to the labor and delivery unit for contractions. The patient states that her last pregnancy was delivered via C-section, but she wants to deliver this one vaginally. She states that she knows the risks and is willing to accept them.*

ROS:
- *Contractions: Present*
- *Fetal movement: Present*
- *Vaginal bleeding: Absent*
- *Leakage of fluid: Present*

PE:
- *Gen: Awake, alert, oriented ×3, mild pain distress*
- *CVS: Normal*
- *Lungs: Clear*
- *Abd: Gravid, contraction present*
- *Ext: 1+ edema bilaterally*

Cervical examination: *7 cm, 100% effaced, -1 station*

Fetal Heart Monitoring: *Reassuring, good variability, + accelerations, no decelerations*

Which of the following is a complication of vaginal birth after C-section (VBAC)?

a. Infection

b. Hemorrhage

c. Pelvic floor damage

d. Uterine rupture

Answer d. Uterine rupture

Uterine rupture is a life-threatening complication in women who undergo VBAC. Infection rates, hemorrhage, and pelvic floor damage do not show a significant increase from C-section to VBAC.

Which uterine scar is most associated with uterine rupture?

a. Classical

b. Low transverse

c. Low vertical

Answer a. Classical incision

Classical incisions have the highest risk of rupture during VBAC.

Move the clock forward 2 hours.

Interval History: *The patient is screaming in pain.*

Fetal Heart Rate: *No fetal heart rate or contractions seen on the monitor*

Cervical Examination: *7 cm, 100% effaced, no fetal head felt*

What is the next step in the management of this patient?

a. Emergent C-section

b. Reposition the fetal monitor

c. Await normal spontaneous vaginal delivery

d. Vacuum-assisted delivery

Answer a. Emergent C-section

This patient is experiencing uterine rupture. Uterine rupture is a clinical diagnosis based on the fetal heart rate and loss of station. The fetus is probably somewhere in the abdomen and no longer in the uterus. That is why the fetal heart rate cannot be seen on the monitor; it is in the wrong spot. Uterine rupture is a life-threatening complication that requires surgical correction and possible cesarean hysterectomy.

Interval History: *An emergency C-Section was done, and the baby was found in the abdomen. A healthy baby boy was born. The uterine rupture could not be repaired, and a hysterectomy was performed.*

CASE 3: Shoulder Dystocia

CC: *"I'm in labor. OUCH!"*

Setting: *Inpatient unit (labor and delivery)*

VS: *BP, 125/88 mm Hg; P, 95 beats/min; R, 12 breaths/min; T, 98.6°F*

HPI: *A 34-year-old G_2P_{1001} with an IUP at 38 weeks' gestation presents to labor and delivery for contractions. The patient states that she has had gestational diabetes that was diet controlled throughout her pregnancy. She states that she has had routine prenatal care.*

ROS:
- *Contractions: Present*
- *Fetal movement: Present*
- *Vaginal bleeding: Absent*
- *Leakage of fluid: Present*

PE:
- *Gen: Awake, alert, oriented ×3, mild pain distress*
- *CVS: S_1S_2+ RRR no m/r/g*
- *Lungs: CTA bilaterally*
- *Abd: Gravid, contractions present*
- *Ext: 1+ edema bilaterally*

Cervical Examination: *7 cm, 100% effaced, -1 station*

Fetal Heart Monitoring: *Reassuring, good variability, accelerations are present, no decelerations*

What is the next step in the management of this patient?

a. Complete blood count (CBC)

b. Finger stick

c. HgbA1C

d. Administer insulin drip

e. Administer Ampicillin

Answer b. Finger stick for blood glucose

All mothers with diabetes who are in labor should have their blood glucose checked. This can be done via a finger stick or a metabolic panel. If the patient's blood sugar is extremely elevated, administration of insulin may be necessary. Without a blood sugar level, insulin use is premature. HgbA1c is a measure of the patient's blood sugar for the past 3 months. This will not show what the sugar is now. CBC may be done, but a finger stick will allow you to further manage the patient. Therefore, if the question states the patient has diabetes, the answer should have something to do with diabetes. Ampicillin and CBC are irrelevant at this time. Ampicillin would be given to mothers who have group B streptococcus on vaginal culture done at 36 weeks' gestation.

Move the clock forward 5 minutes.

Interval History: *Finger stick returns as 140 mg/dL.*

What is the patient at risk for?

a. Placental abruption
b. Placenta previa
c. Preeclampsia

d. Shoulder dystocia
e. Uterine rupture

Answer d. Shoulder dystocia

Shoulder dystocia is a common complication in mothers with diabetes. Shoulder dystocia occurs during delivery when the anterior shoulder becomes stuck behind the pubis symphysis. Shoulder dystocia is common in mothers with diabetes because the baby is large or macrosomic. When the fetus is large, there is an increased risk for shoulder dystocia.

Move the clock forward 2 hours.

Interval History: *The patient states that she feels like pushing. Cervical examination done at that time shows a fully dilated cervix, 100% effacement, and -1 station. The mother starts to push and is moved to the delivery room.*

Upon delivery of the head of the baby, the baby gets stuck. The patient is pushing, but the baby cannot be delivered.

What is the next step in the management of this patient?

a. Delivery of the anterior shoulder
b. Delivery of the posterior shoulder
c. Fracture the clavicle

d. McRobert's maneuver
e. Zavanelli maneuver

Answer d. McRobert's maneuver

Shoulder dystocia occurs when the fetal head has been delivered but the rest of the body is stuck. The fetal anterior shoulder is stuck behind the pubis symphysis. The first step in management is McRobert's maneuver (see Figure 7-19). In this maneuver, the mother will reach and pull her legs to her chest. This will open up the pelvis. The second part to the maneuver includes suprapubic pressure to push the baby's shoulder under the pubis symphysis. If McRobert's maneuver does not relieve the shoulder dystocia, then delivery of the posterior shoulder should be done. By delivering the posterior shoulder, this will drop the anterior shoulder and relieve the obstruction. These two maneuvers will successfully deliver most shoulder dystocias. However, if these do not, the next step would be fracturing of the clavicle. Zavanelli maneuver is the last step in the treatment of shoulder dystocia and has high mortality rate for both the mother and baby. The Zavanelli maneuver includes pushing the fetal head back into the mother and then doing an emergency C-section.

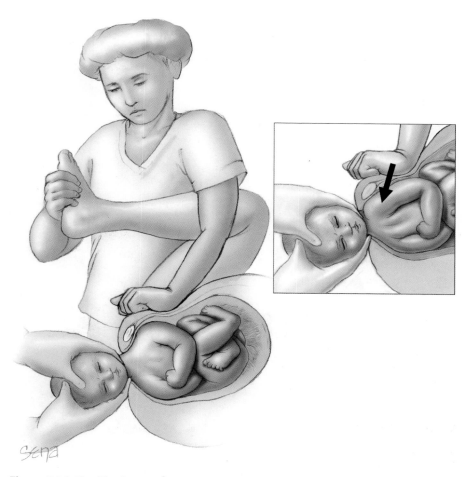

Figure 7-19. Shoulder dystocia. (Reproduced with permission from Cunningham F, Leveno K, Bloom S, et al. *Williams Obstetrics,* 23rd ed. New York: McGraw-Hill; 2010).

Interval History: *McRobert's maneuver was successful, and a baby boy was delivered.*

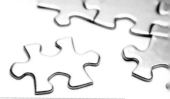

CHAPTER 8

POSTPARTUM PROBLEMS

CASE 1: Postpartum Bleeding

CC: *"I gave birth and wont stop bleeding."*

Setting: *Inpatient unit (labor and delivery)*

VS: *BP, 120/75 mm Hg; P, 95 beats/min; R, 12 breaths/min; T, 98.6°F*

HPI: *A 27-year-old woman with an intrauterine pregnancy at 39 weeks' gestation presented in active labor. The patient became fully dilated and delivered a baby boy 5 minutes ago. The patient then delivered the placenta without complication. There were no lacerations visualized of the cervix, vagina, or vulva. However, the patient is continuing to bleed.*

What is the next step in the management of this patient?

a. Administer oxytocin

b. Administer methylergonovine

c. Administer blood products

d. Perform bimanual uterine massage

e. Perform hysterectomy

Answer d. Perform bimanual uterine massage

The first step in postpartum hemorrhage after a vaginal delivery is to do a bimanual uterine massage (Figure 8-1). The most common reason for postpartum hemorrhage is uterine atony. If the patient continued to bleed after bimanual massage, administration of oxytocin and methylergonovine may be necessary. Blood products and hysterectomy are given later. Hysterectomy is done if oxytocin and methylergonovine cannot control the bleeding and the hematocrit continues to drop.

Methylergonovine causes vasoconstriction of uterine vessels.

Uterine atony = Uterus not contracting after delivery
Atony means: A = Without tony = Contraction

Risk factors for uterine atony:
• Overdistention
• Infection
• Uterine inversion
• Retained placenta

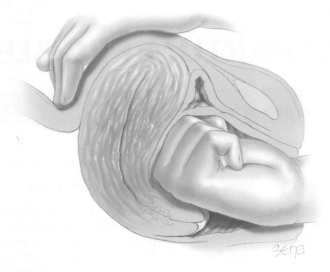

Figure 8-1. Bimanual massage. (Reproduced with permission from Cunningham F, Leveno K, Bloom S, et al. *Williams Obstetrics,* 23rd ed. New York: McGraw-Hill; 2010.)

Move the clock forward 5 minutes.

Interval History: *Despite bimanual massage and an increase in oxytocin, the patient continues to have vaginal bleeding.*

What should be checked before the administration of methylergonovine?

a. Blood pressure

b. Cranial nerves

c. Pulse

d. Pulse oximeter

Answer a. Blood pressure

Methylergonovine is an uterotonic drug that causes vasospasm. It is contraindicated in patients who have hypertension, Raynaud phenomenon, or scleroderma. Patients with coronary artery disease may experience chest pain and myocardial infarction from vasospasm. Methylergonovine may be given every 2 to 4 hours if bleeding does not stop. If the patient does not have a good response during the first administration, a different drug should be chosen. Other uterotonic drugs include carboprost, misoprostol, and carbetocin; these are all possible second-line drugs.

Move the clock forward 5 minutes.

Interval History: *Vital signs were taken and return as BP, 150/90 mm Hg; P, 80 beats/min; R, 16 breaths/min; and T, 98.6°F.*

The patient is continuing to bleed vaginally despite an increase in oxytocin and bimanual massage. Physical examination does not reveal cervical, labial, or vulvar lacerations. No uterine inversion is noted. The placenta was delivered intact.

What is the next step in the management of this patient?

a. Administer methylergonovine

b. Administer oxytocin

c. Administer carboprost

d. Administer Misoprostol

Answer d. Administer misoprostol

This patient is experiencing a postpartum hemorrhage and has hypertension. Hypertension is a contraindication to both methylergonovine and carboprost. If the patient is not responding to an increased dose of oxytocin, administering it again will not help. Misoprostol is the drug of choice in women with hypertension and postpartum hemorrhage. Uterotonic drugs are used to induce contractions; uterine contractions cause constriction not only of the muscles but also of the vessels, causing a decrease in bleeding.

Carboprost:
- Prostaglandin F2 analog
- Increases myometrial contraction
- Expels products of conception
- Decreases bleeding

Misoprostol:
- Prostaglandin E1 analog
- Induces uterine contractions
- Induces labor
- Medical termination of pregnancy

After administration of misoprostol, the uterine bleeding stopped.

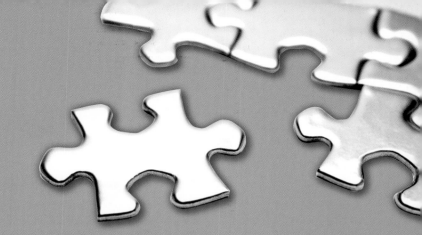

SECTION II
Gynecology

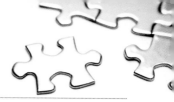

CHAPTER 9

UTERINE ABNORMALITIES

CASE 1: Fibroids

CC: *"My menstruation is long and heavy."*

Setting: *Outpatient office*

VS: *BP, 110/70 mm Hg; P, 95 beats/min; R, 17 breaths/min; T, 98.6°F*

HPI: *A 27-year-old African American woman presents with several months of prolonged menstrual bleeding and increased volume of menstrual flow. She also has a sensation of heaviness in her abdomen. She denies abdominal pain, nausea, vomiting, diarrhea, and constipation. She fatigues easily.*

PE:
- *Gen: Awake, alert, oriented ×3, no acute distress*
- *CVS: Regular rate and rhythm, no murmurs, rubs, or gallops*
- *Lungs: Clear to auscultation bilaterally*
- *Abd: Soft, nontender, nondistended, + bowel sounds*
- *Pelvis: Cervix appears normal, no cervical motion tenderness, no adnexal masses felt*

What is the term for what this patient is experiencing?

a. Amenorrhea

b. Dysmenorrhea

c. Menorrhagia

d. Metrorrhagia

e. Polymenorrhea

Answer c. Menorrhagia

Term	Definition
Amenorrhea	Absence of menstruation for three cycles
Dysmenorrhea	Painful menstruation
Menorrhagia	Prolonged or excessive menstrual bleeding
Metrorrhagia	Less menstrual bleeding at irregular cycles
Polymenorrhea	Menstruation that occurs at less than every 24 days
Dysfunctional uterine bleeding	Unexplained abnormal bleeding
Postcoital bleeding	Bleeding after sex

Postcoital bleeding is cervical pathology until proven otherwise.

Dysfunctional uterine bleeding:
• Anovulatory bleeding
• Diagnosis of exclusion
• Bleeding occurs when the endometrium outgrows its blood supply

Which of the following is the next step in the management of this patient?

a. Hysteroscopy

b. Hysterosalpingography

c. Magnetic resonance imaging (MRI)

d. Ultrasonography (US)

Answer d. Ultrasonography (US)

This patient most likely has "fibroids," or leiomyoma of the uterus. Leiomyomas are the most common benign tumor of the uterus. US is the preferred method of diagnosis for its accessibility and sensitivity (Figure 9-1). Hysterosalpingography can identify any abnormalities in the contour of the endometrial cavity, but cannot identify any abnormality that is unconnected with the endometrial lining. Hysteroscopy is a more invasive procedure that involves placing a scope into the uterus. This may be done after US; however, noninvasive tests are always preferred. MRI can distinguish among leiomyoma, leiomyosarcoma, and adenomyosis. MRI is not a screening test and is generally used for surgical planning.

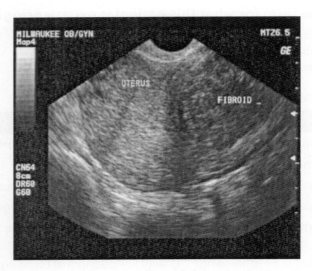

Figure 9-1. Ultrasound image of leiomyomas (fibroids). (Reproduced with permission from DeCherney AH. *Current Diagnosis & Treatment,* 11th ed. New York: McGraw-Hill; 2013.)

On the CCS, initial orders include complete blood count (CBC), prothrombin time and activated partial thromboplastin time (aPTT), and US.

Transabdominal US is done first; transvaginal US is done if transabdominal is unrevealing.

Risk factors for leiomyomas:
- African American
- Nulliparity
- Family history
- Hypertension

What kind of tissue makes up a leiomyoma?

a. Glandular tissue
b. Smooth muscle
c. Striated muscle
d. Fibrous connective tissue
e. Loose connective tissue

Answer b. Smooth muscle

Leiomyomas are composed of smooth muscle of the myometrium. There are several types of leiomyomas depending on the location of the benign tumor (Figure 9-2).

Name	Location
Intermural	Inside myometrial wall
Submucosal	Just under the surface of the endometrium; often protrude into the endometrial cavity
Subserosal	Just under the serosal surface of the uterus; often protrude into the abdominal cavity
Cervical	As name states, in the cervix
Pendulated	Has a stalk that is connected to the uterus
Intercavitary	Inside the uterine cavity

How does estrogen increase the growth of leiomyomas?

a. Stimulates growth hormone
b. Interferes with apoptosis
c. Stimulates proliferation of smooth muscle cells
d. Decreases luteinizing hormone (LH) and follicle-stimulating hormone (FSH) levels

Answer c. Stimulates proliferation of smooth muscle cells

Estrogen stimulates proliferation of smooth muscle cells. Progesterone interferes with apoptosis, allowing the leiomyoma to grow. Increased growth factors stimulate production of fibronectin.

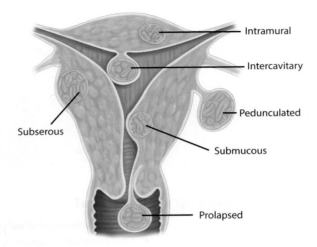

Figure 9-2. Types of leiomyomas. (Reproduced with permission from Brunicardi FC. *Schwartz's Principles of Surgery*, 9th ed. New York: McGraw-Hill; 2010.)

Fibroid growth depends on estrogen and progesterone.

Apoptosis = Programmed cell death (Figure 9-3)

Fibroids tend to outgrow the blood supply in pregnancy and become painful.

Adenomyosis = Endometrial glands and stroma in the myometrium
• Same presentation as fibroids
• "Globular" uterus on physical examination (diffuse enlargement)
• Only definitive diagnosis and treatment is hysterectomy

Move the clock forward 2 weeks.

Lab Results:
• *CBC: Hematocrit 28%*   • *Prothrombin time/aPTT: Normal*

US: *Intermural and submucosal leiomyoma*

Interval History: *The patient continues to have pain and prolonged menstruation.*

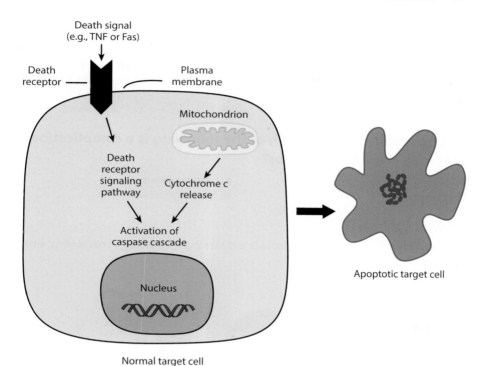

Figure 9-3. Apoptosis. Extracellular pathway initiated by activation of tumor necrosis factor (TNF) or Fas leads to activation of the caspase pathway. The intracellular pathway is initiated by release of cytochrome C from the mitochondria. Apoptosis causes destruction of the DNA into fragments and membranes and eventual digestion by other cells. (Reproduced with permission from Brunicardi FC. *Schwartz's Principles of Surgery,* 9th ed. New York: McGraw-Hill; 2010.)

What is the next step in the management of this patient?

a. Repeat US in 6 months
b. Hysterectomy
c. Uterine artery embolization

d. Intrauterine device
e. Myomectomy
f. Oral contraceptive pills (OCPs)

Answer f. Oral contraceptive pills (OCPs)

OCPs are the first-line treatment for leiomyomas. In general, OCPs will decrease the amount of blood loss monthly, helping to prevent anemia. However, they will not help with the sensation of fullness in her abdomen. Repeating the US in 6 months would be the option if this patient was asymptomatic. Hysterectomy and uterine artery embolization are reserved for women who are no longer of childbearing age or have completed their families. Myomectomy is the surgical option for this patient who is of childbearing age. Myomectomy means taking out the muscular "bump" in the uterus while still trying to leave the rest of the uterus intact. Intrauterine devices are contraindicated when there are submucosal leiomyomas because they distort the endometrial cavity.

> *Move the clock forward 3 months*
>
> **Interval History:** *The patient used OCPs for several months but is still experiencing significant pressure in her lower abdomen. She would now like to explore her surgical options. She would like to have children.*

After a myomectomy, which of the following is a complication that may occur during labor?

a. Preterm labor

b. Uterine atony

c. Uterine rupture

d. No complications

Answer c. Uterine rupture

The risk factors for uterine rupture include any manipulation of the uterus such as myomectomy (Figure 9-4).

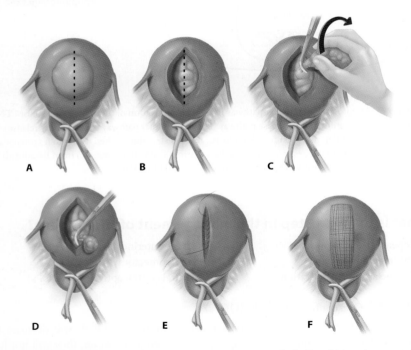

Figure 9-4. Myomectomy. Step **A-F** are the surgical steps in removal of a fibroid. Note that surgical scars on the uterus increase the risk for uterine rupture during childbirth. (Reproduced with permission from Brunicardi FC. *Schwartz's Principles of Surgery*, 9th ed. New York: McGraw-Hill; 2010.)

> *The patient was informed of the risks and benefits and would like to consider her options.*

CASE 2: Endometriosis

CC: *"I can't get pregnant."*

Setting: *Outpatient office*

VS: *BP, 120/80 mm Hg; P, 82 beats/min; R, 16 breaths/min; T, 97.8°F; body mass index (BMI), 24*

HPI: *A 26-year-old woman G_0P_0 presents to the office for infertility. The patient states that she and her husband have been trying to conceive for almost 2 years without success. She menstruates regularly. Her cycles occur every 28 days with 5 or 6 days of bleeding. She does have some pain during menstruation but not more than usual. She has no medical, surgical, or sexually transmitted disease. The patient and her husband have sexual relations during ovulation on a daily basis. She has had multiple blood tests by her primary care provider (PCP), all of which are normal.*

ROS: *Negative*

PE:
- *Gen: Awake, alert, oriented ×3, no acute distress*
- *CVS: Normal*
- *Lungs: Normal*
- *Abd: Soft, nontender, nondistended, +bowel sounds*
- *Pelvic exam: Within normal limits*

Which of the following is most useful?

a. Prolactin level

b. Glucose level

c. Growth hormone level

d. Imaging study of the pelvis

e. Cortisol level

Answer a. Prolactin level

Hyperprolactinemia is a cause of infertility. Abnormally high prolactin levels inhibit ovulation. This is the mechanism of why breastfeeding after pregnancy inhibits ovulation and prevents conception during breastfeeding. High prolactin levels also cause galactorrhea in women.

Prolactin's effect on the hypothalamus and pituitary:
- Inhibition of LH and FSH surge
- Inhibition of gonadotropin-releasing hormone
- No LH surge = No ovulation

What is the next step in the management?

a. Endometrial biopsy

b. Semen analysis

c. Postcoital test

d. Laparoscopy

e. Hysterosalpingography

Answer b. Semen analysis

The first step in the evaluation of infertility is a thorough evaluation of the history and physical examination findings. Often the problem is not enough sexual activity at the right time in the menstrual cycle, history of menstrual irregularity, or sexual dysfunction. Remember, a patient can say, "We are having lots of sex" but not know that ovulation is in the middle of the cycle. Make sure to ask about the duration of infertility. Infertility as a medical diagnosis does not mean failing to conceive for just 1 or 2 months. Patients should be trying for at least 1 year before doing an infertility evaluation.

The PCP should order thyroid-stimulating hormone (TSH), prolactin, LH, FSH, estrogen, progesterone, and testosterone levels. If they are within normal limits, as stated in this question, the next step is semen analysis. Semen analysis is done after 7 to 10 days of abstinence. Semen analysis will include a sperm count, sperm morphology, sperm motility, pH of the semen, white blood cell (WBC) count, and fructose level. Endometrial biopsy and postcoital tests are not recommended in the evaluation of infertility. Hysterosalpingography and laparoscopy are both invasive and therefore never the first-line diagnostic test. They might be done later if the initial tests are unrevealing.

Move the clock forward 1 week.

Interval History: *The patient and her husband continue to try to have a baby. Semen results are normal. Hormone levels are within normal limits.*

What is the next step in the management of this patient?

a. Laparoscopy

b. Hysterosalpingography

c. Tell them to have more sex

d. Basal body temperature charting

Answer b. Hysterosalpingography

Hysterosalpingography is a test of the patency of the woman's fallopian tubes (Figure 9-5). In hysterosalpingography, a small amount of dye is injected through the cervix into the uterus. Fluoroscopy is done while the dye is injected to monitor the shape of the uterus and to see if the dye is expressed or travels through the fallopian tubes. If the dye is expressed, the fallopian tubes are patent or open. At least one fallopian tube must be patent to conceive. The sperm need to have access to the fallopian tubes to fertilize the egg. The results of a hysterosalpingography may also show structural abnormalities in the uterus. Laparoscopy is a surgical intervention and would be the final step in the management of this patient. Charting the basal body temperature lacks meaningful precision. When the patients have already been trying for 1 year, telling them to have more sex will not be effective.

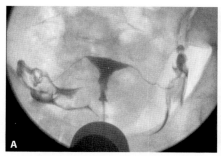

Normal

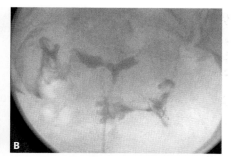

Asherman syndrome

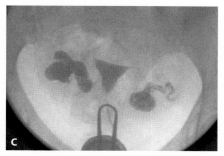

Bilateral hydrosalpinges

Figure 9-5. Hysterosalpingogram. **A,** Normal. Dye is extricated from the fallopian tubes and shows normal contour of the uterus. **B,** Asherman syndrome: irregularly shaped endometrial cavity. **C,** Hydrosalpinges, fallopian tube dilation. (Photos contributed by Dr. Kevin Doody and used with permission from Hoffman BL, Schorge J, Halvorson L, et al (eds). *Williams Gynecology,* 2nd ed. New York: McGraw-Hill; 2012.)

Interval History: *Hysterosalpingography shows a normal contour (shape) and size of the uterus, as well as patent fallopian tubes. The patient is still unable to conceive.*
Laparoscopy is done and shows moderate endometriosis. Surgical intervention to remove the endometriomas is performed.

What is the next step in the management of this patient?

a. Await natural pregnancy
b. Start clomiphene

c. Start oral contraceptive pills
d. Start Danazol

Answer a. Await natural pregnancy.

The patient underwent laparoscopy, which showed endometriosis. Endometriosis is the growth of endometrium outside the endometrial cavity. This may present as infertility, dysmenorrhea, or dyspareunia or may be asymptomatic. After a laparoscopic intervention, the patient should try to conceive naturally for 6 months. After this period, clomiphene may be started. OCPs are the medical treatment for endometriosis. Because the patient underwent surgical treatment, medical treatment is not necessary at this time. Besides, the patient's ultimate goal is to get pregnant. Placing the patient on birth control would be the opposite of what the patient wants.

GnRH agonists are superior to Danazol for endometriosis treatment. Danazol is an androgen analog. Giving an androgen will not help infertility. Danazol is used in the medical management of pain associated with endometriosis. Endometriosis is stimulated by estrogens. Androgens should block that effect.

Endometriosis:
• Endometrial glands outside the uterus (Figure 9-6)

Endometriosis symptoms:
• Infertility
• Dysmenorrhea (painful periods)
• Dyspareunia (painful sex)
• Abnormal menstrual bleeding

Endometriosis treatment:
• Medical
   · OCPs
   · GnRH agonists (Leuprolide, Goserelin, Nafarelin)
   · Danazol (androgen analog)
   · Progestin
• Surgical

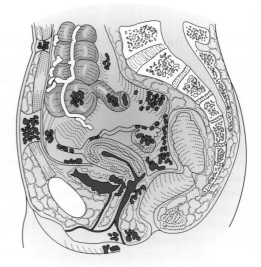

Figure 9-6. Location of possible endometriomas. (Reproduced with permission from Way LW. *Current Surgical Diagnosis & Treatment*, 7th ed. Lange, McGraw-Hill; 1985.)

GnRH agonists:
- Initial bump up in LH and FSH
- Downregulation of pituitary receptors
- Shutting off of both LH and FSH

Interval History: *Three months later, the couple returns for amenorrhea. The patient was found to be pregnant with twins.*

CASE 3: Postmenopausal Bleeding

CC: *"I'm having vaginal bleeding."*

Setting: *Outpatient office*

VS: *BP, 135/80 mm Hg; P, 76 beats/min; R, 18 breaths/min; T, 98.9°F*

HPI: *A 65-year-old woman with PMH of hypertension treated with lisinopril and hydro-chlorothiazide (HCTZ) presents to the office for vaginal bleeding. The bleeding started last month. It was lighter than her menstruation used to be and lasted for 4 days.*

ROS:
• *No fever, chills, or weight loss*
• *No chest pain or shortness of breath*
• *No abdominal pain, nausea, vomiting, diarrhea, constipation, or distention*

PE:
• *Gen: Awake, alert, oriented ×3, no acute distress*
• *CVS: S_1S_2 + RRR no m/r/g*
• *Lungs: CTA bilaterally*
• *Abd: Soft, nontender, nondistended, + bowel sounds*
• *Ext: No edema*
• *Pelvic: Cervix appears normal, no lacerations seen, bimanual examination findings within normal limits*

What is the next step in the management of this patient?

a. Transabdominal US
b. Endometrial biopsy

c. No further management is needed
d. CT scan

Answer b. Endometrial biopsy

Endometrial biopsy is done as an initial test in all women with postmenopausal bleeding who do not have an identifiable lesion on their cervix (Figure 9-7). Endometrial carcinoma is responsible for almost 10% of postmenopausal bleeding patients. Other common causes include endometrial polyps and atrophy of the endometrium or vagina.

Postmenopausal bleeding = Endometrial biopsy

Interval History: *The endometrial biopsy shows endometrial carcinoma. US shows mild invasion of the myometrium. The patient will be referred to a gynecologic oncologist.*

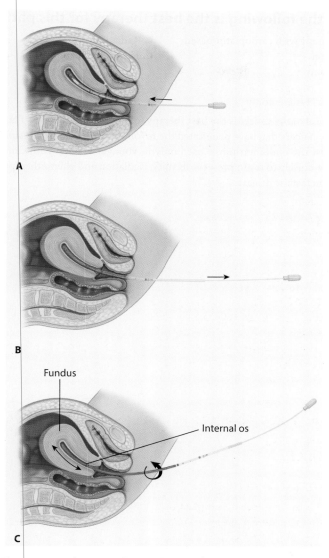

Figure 9-7. The steps to perform an endometrial biopsy. (Reproduced with permission from Hoffman BL, Schorge J, Halvorson L, et al (eds). *Williams Gynecology,* 2nd ed. New York: McGraw-Hill; 2012.)

Consultants do not give advice or recommendations on step 3 CCS. Ask for them anyway to show you know when you need help.

Which of the following is the best therapy for this patient?

a. Chemotherapy with carboplatin-based combination

b. Hysterectomy

c. Radiation

d. Hormonal manipulation

Answer b. Hysterectomy

Surgical removal of the cancer is the best therapy for endometrial cancer. This is especially important for cancers that have penetrated the myometrium. Hormonal manipulation and removal of just the endometrium is used only in younger women with cancer that does not invade the muscle to try to preserve fertility. Radiation and chemotherapy are used for recurrent or metastatic disease.

CHAPTER 10

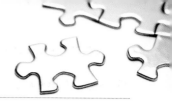

PREGNANCY PREVENTION AND SEXUALLY TRANSMITTED INFECTIONS

CASE 1: Contraception

CC: *"I need birth control."*

Setting: *Outpatient office*

VS: *BP, 110/70 mm Hg; P, 82 beats/min; R, 16 breaths/min; T, 98.5°F*

HPI: *A 14-year-old young woman with no PMH, no PSH presents to the office stating that she would like to begin birth control. She is sexually active with multiple male partners. Her last menstrual period (LMP) was 3 weeks ago.*

ROS: *No fever, chills, abdominal pain, nausea, vomiting, diarrhea, constipation, chest pain, shortness of breath, history of pulmonary embolism, or medical problems*

PE:
- *Gen: Awake, alert, oriented ×3, no acute distress*
- *CVS: S_1S_2 + RRR no m/r/g*
- *Lungs: CTA bilaterally*
- *Abd: Soft, nontender, nondistended, + bowel sounds*
- *Ext: no edema*

Which of the following is the next step in the management of this patient?

a. CBC

b. CMP

c. Cervical cultures

d. Urine beta-human chorionic gonadotropin (BHCG)

Answer d. Urine beta-human chorionic gonadotropin (BHCG)

Women of childbearing age need to have a BHCG level before starting birth control. Patients should start their birth control after their next menstrual period.

On the CCS, the initial order set would include BHCG and vaginal swabs.

But wait! This patient is only 14! What is the recommendation regarding birth control in minors?

a. Must get parental consent
b. Patient does not need parental consent

c. Only if patient had a child, then she could consent to her own birth control
d. Patient is emancipated

Answer b. Patient does not need parental consent

Pediatric patients are defined as those younger than 18 years old. Minors need to have parental consent for all medical treatments with the exception of sexually transmitted diseases (STDs), birth control, prenatal care, or substance abuse treatment. Minors become fully emancipated when they are married *and* self-supporting *or* in the military. A fully emancipated minor can consent to any procedure.

> **Interval History:** *After discussion about all of the different types of contraception, the patient decides that she would like an intrauterine device (IUD).*

Which of the following should be done before insertion?

a. Cervical cultures and Chlamydia serology
b. Pap smear

c. Transvaginal ultrasonography (US)
d. Nothing needs to be done

Answer a. Cervical swabs and Chlamydia serology

Cervical swabs or nucleic acid amplification testing (NAAT) for gonorrhea and Chlamydia are recommended before insertion of the IUD. A Pap smear is not recommended regardless of sexual activity until age 21 years.

Overview of the different types of contraception (Figure 10-1):

Type of Contraception	Pros	Cons
Female condoms	Protect against HIV and other STDs	Larger and bulkier than male condoms
Male condoms	Easy to use; protect against HIV/STD	Dependent on male use
Oral contraceptive pills (OCPs)	Most common; regulate menstruation Reduce the risk of ovarian cancer, endometrial cancer, and ectopic pregnancy	Do not protect against HIV and other STDs; must take on a daily basis; increased risk of DVT and PE

(Continued)

Type of Contraception	Pros	Cons
Vaginal ring	Easy to use; same problems as OCPs	Does not protect against HIV or other STDs; increased risk of DVT and PE
Transdermal patch	Place on skin for 1 week; then remove and replace with a new one Same problems as OCPs	Same cons as OCPs Weekly, not daily
Intrauterine device	Placed in uterus; good for 5–10 years	Does not protect against HIV and other STDs Associated with PID when placed
Sterilization	Permanent	Increased risk of ectopic pregnancy with tubal ligation

DVT, deep vein thrombosis; PID, pelvic inflammatory disease; PE, pulmonary embolism; STD, sexually transmitted disease.

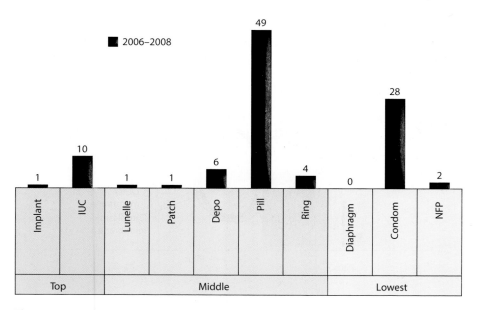

Figure 10-1. Effectiveness of birth control types. IUC, intrauterine contraception; NFP, natural family planning. (Reproduced with permission from Hoffman BL, Schorge J, Halvorson L, et al (eds). *Williams Gynecology*, 2nd ed. New York: McGraw-Hill; 2012.)

Move the clock forward 1 week.

Interval History: *Cervical cultures were done and are positive for gonorrhea (Figures 10-2 and 10-3). The patient returns for follow-up. She is feeling well and has no vaginal discharge. The patient denies vaginal pruritus.*

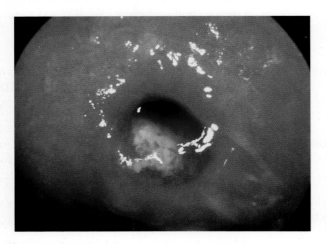

Figure 10-2. Cervicitis with gonorrhea. (Photo contributed by King K. Holmes and used with permission from Handsfield HH. *Color Atlas and Synopsis of Sexually Transmitted Diseases.* New York: McGraw-Hill; 1992.)

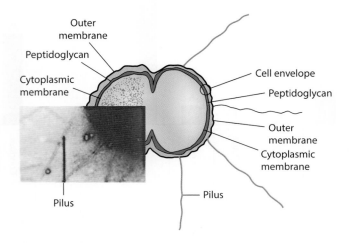

Figure 10-3. Gonorrhea with pili and three-layer cell envelope. (Reproduced with permission from Brooks GF, Carroll KC, Butel J, Morse S. *Jawetz, Melnick, & Adelberg's Medical Microbiology,* 26th ed. New York: McGraw-Hill; 2013.)

Which is the treatment for this patient?

a. Azithromycin alone
b. Azithromycin plus doxycycline

c. Azithromycin plus ceftriaxone
d. Ceftriaxone alone

Answer c. Azithromycin plus ceftriaxone

Even though the culture grew *Neisseria gonorrhea,* treatment should be given for both gonorrhea and Chlamydia. When gonorrhea is present, there is Chlamydia co-infection in as many as 50% of patients. Therefore, if gonorrhea is present, Chlamydia should be treated for as well. Ceftriaxone is for gonorrhea, and azithromycin is for Chlamydia. Azithromycin and doxycycline can both be used to treat Chlamydia.

Gonorrhea grows on chocolate agar (Thayer Martin media). This media has the following antibiotics.
• Vancomycin kills gram-positive competition.
• Colistin kills gram negatives but not gonorrhea.
• Nystatin kills fungi.

Interval History: *Treatment was implemented, and after consideration, the patient chose to use the vaginal ring for contraception. The patient should return yearly for NAAT testing for Chlamydia, as recommended by the U.S. Preventive Services Task Force (USPSTF), until age 24 years.*

CASE 2: Sexually Transmitted Infections

CC: *"I have vaginal discharge."*

Setting: *Outpatient office*

VS: *BP, 120/80 mm Hg; P, 82 beats/min; R, 14 breaths/min; T, 98.6°F*

HPI: 25-year-old G_2P_{0020} with no PMH presents to the office for vaginal discharge and itching. She has been sexually active with 3 partners in the last month. She does not always use condoms. The vaginal discharge started about 1 week ago and is profuse and green. She does not describe it as malodorous. Her LMP was last week.

Terminology of gravida (G) and parity (P):
- G = Total number of pregnancies
- P = **F**ull term, **p**remature, **a**bortions, **l**ive children

---

ROS:
- *Denies fever and chills*
- *Denies chest pain, shortness of breath, abdominal pain, nausea, vomiting, diarrhea, and constipation*

PE:
- *Gen: Awake, alert, oriented ×3, no acute distress*
- *CVS: S_1S_2 + RRR no m/r/g*
- *Lungs: CTA bilaterally*
- *Abd: Soft, nontender, nondistended, + bowel sounds*

Vaginal Exam: *Cervix appears red and irritated; profuse green vaginal discharge*

Bimanual Exam: *No cervical motion tenderness (CMT); no adnexal tenderness or enlargement*

Which of the following is the next step in the management of this patient?

a. Administer ceftriaxone and azithromycin

b. Administer fluconazole

c. Administer metronidazole

d. Potassium hydroxide (KOH) and wet prep

e. No further treatment is necessary

f. Vaginal culture

Answer d. Potassium hydroxide (KOH) and wet prep

Diagnostic tests should always be done before a patient is treated for vaginitis or cervicitis. This is because you cannot tell the difference among bacterial vaginitis, fungal vaginitis, and trichomonas without testing. Take the cultures and KOH and then treat what is found. The KOH shows fungi. The wet mount is both for the clue cells of bacterial vaginitis as well as the freely motile forms of trichomoniasis. Vaginal culture can be misleading. The vagina is home to numerous organisms, and most are nonpathogenic.

Vaginal culture is the most common wrong answer. The KOH and wet mount office or ambulatory clinic–based tests are instantly available. The NAAT on a swab is the most precise test for gonorrhea and Chlamydia.

Initial Order set for CCS: Vaginal swab for NAAT for gonorrhea and Chlamydia, saline wet mount and KOH wet prep, and vaginal pH.

Normal vaginal pH <4.5
Lactobacillus make a normal vaginal pH
Low pH prevents abnormal bacterial overgrowth

Move the clock forward 1 hour.

Interval History: *Wet prep and KOH were done in the office: Wet prep shows motile organisms under the microscope (Figure 10-4).*

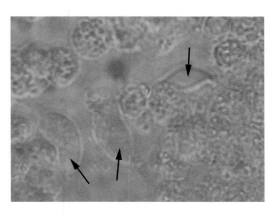

pH < 4.5 - candidasis
   >4.5 - bacterial vaginosis
      or
   trichomoniasis

Figure 10-4. *Trichomonas (arrows).* (Reproduced with permission from Richard P. Usatine.)

What is the treatment of choice?

a. Ceftriaxone and azithromycin for the patient

b. Ceftriaxone and azithromycin for the patient and partner

c. Fluconazole for the patient

d. Fluconazole for the patient and partner

e. Metronidazole for the patient

f. Metronidazole for the patient and partner

Answer f. Metronidazole for the patient and partner

The most likely infection in this patient is with *Trichomonas* spp. It presents with profuse, green, and frothy vaginal discharge. On wet prep, motile organisms are seen. Treatment for *Trichomonas* infection is metronidazole for the patient and her partner.

Other types of vaginitis:

Type of Vaginitis	Bacteria	Symptom	Test	Treatment
Candida albicans (yeast infection)	*C. albicans* (Figure 10-5)	Cheesy white vaginal discharge	Pseudohyphae on KOH prep	Antifungal creams or oral antifungal
Bacterial vaginosis	*Gardnerella*	Gray or white vaginal discharge with fishy odor	KOH shows clue cells	Metronidazole for patient only
Trichomonas	*Trichomonas vaginalis* (Figure 10-6)	Profuse, green, frothy discharge	KOH shows motile flagellates	Metronidazole for the patient and partner

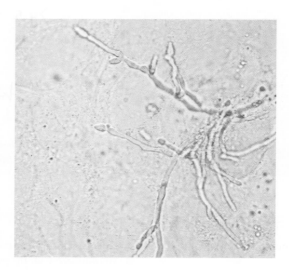

Figure 10-5. *Candida* on potassium hydroxide (KOH) wet mount. (Used with permission of David A. Eschenbach, MD and reproduced with permission from Handsfield HH. *Color Atlas and Synopsis of Sexually Transmitted Diseases.* New York: McGraw-Hill; 1992.)

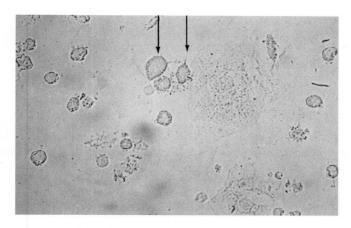

Figure 10-6. *Trichomonas* (*arrows*). (Reproduced with permission from Handsfield HH. *Atlas of Sexually Transmitted Diseases.* New York: McGraw-Hill; 1992.)

CASE 3: Cervicitis

CC: *"I'm here for my annual exam."*

Setting: *Outpatient office*

VS: *BP, 125/75 mm Hg; P, 78 beats/min; R, 16 breaths/min; T, 98.4°F*

HPI: *A 23-year-old woman with no PMH presents to the office for her annual gynecologic examination. She has never been pregnant. She has had five lifetime partners. She does not have vaginal discharge, vaginal pruritus, or dyspareunia. Her menstruation is regular every 28 days and lasts for 5 days.*

In addition to the Pap smear, what else is indicated?

a. Chlamydia testing
b. Herpes testing

c. Hepatitis testing
d. Trichomonas testing

Answer a. Chlamydia testing

The USPSTF recommends annual screening for Chlamydia in women age 24 years and younger, pregnant women, and women at increased risk (Figure 10-7). Chlamydia infections are often asymptomatic in women or may cause cervicitis. Cervicitis causes vaginal discharge, abnormal vaginal bleeding, or abnormal discharge from the cervix seen on examination. If the infection persists, it may cause pelvic inflammatory disease (PID) and eventually infertility. Chlamydia screening is done in conjunction with gonorrhea and the Pap smear. Herpes, hepatitis, and trichomonas are not routinely screened for during the annual examination.

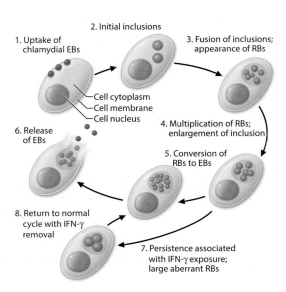

Figure 10-7. Chlamydia life cycle. EB, elementary body; IFN, interferon; RB, reticular body. (Reproduced with permission from Longo DL, Fauci A, Kasper D, et al. *Harrison's Principles of Internal Medicine*, 18th ed, vol. 1. New York: McGraw-Hill; 2011.)

Chlamydia screening is done with NAAT testing.

Chlamydia screening is routinely done:
• Yearly when sexually active until 24 years old
• Pregnant
• Yearly after age 24 years if at increased risk

Risk factors for Chlamydia:
• History of infection
• Multiple sexual partners
• New sexual partners
• Unmarried
• Unprotected intercourse
• History of sexually transmitted infection (any)

Move the clock forward 1 week.

Interval History: *Chlamydia testing returns positive. The patient continues to be asymptomatic. She denies having a current sexual partner.*

What treatments is indicated?

a. Azithromycin

c. Levofloxacin

b. Ceftriaxone

d. Amoxicillin

Answer a. Azithromycin

Azithromycin is the drug of choice in Chlamydia infections. Ceftriaxone is the drug of choice for gonorrhea. If the patient has Chlamydia, there is no need to treat for gonorrhea. However, if gonorrhea is present, concomitant treatment for Chlamydia is warranted. Levofloxacin and amoxicillin may be given if the patient is allergic to azithromycin. However, azithromycin is superior and should be given if able. Quinolones are considered an alternative to azithromycin or doxycycline. Quinolones are not to be used as primary therapy.

Both the patient and the partner must be treated.

How long should the patient abstain from sexual activity after treatment?

a. May be sexually active right away
b. 2 days
c. 5 days

d. 7 days
e. 10 days

Answer d. 7 days

Both the patient and the partner should be treated with azithromycin. They should wait 7 days before resuming sexual activity to prevent reinfection.

When is a test of cure needed?

a. In all women
b. In all men

c. Women treated with azithromycin
d. Pregnant women

Answer d. Pregnant women

All patients with Chlamydia do **not** need a test of cure. Only the following groups of people need a test of cure:

• Pregnant women
• Symptomatic
• Treated with penicillin or cephalosporins

Test of cure should be performed 3 weeks after antibiotic therapy is completed.

CASE 4: Pelvic Inflammatory Disease or Abscess

CC: *"I have pelvic pain."*

Setting: *Outpatient office*

VS: *BP, 125/80 mm Hg; P, 75 beats/min; R, 18 breaths/min; T, 100.5°F*

A 28-year-old woman presents with lower abdominal pain that is worse with intercourse. She had unprotected sex several weeks ago. Her LMP was 2 weeks ago. She denies fever, chills, and vaginal discharge. She takes oral contraception for birth control.

ROS:
- *Abdominal pain present in lower quadrants*
- *Denies nausea, vomiting, diarrhea, or constipation*

PE: *Abdominal tenderness most pronounced in lower quadrants*
- *Copious amounts of green vaginal discharge (Figure 10-8)*
- *Cervical motion tenderness is present*
- *No adnexal enlargement*

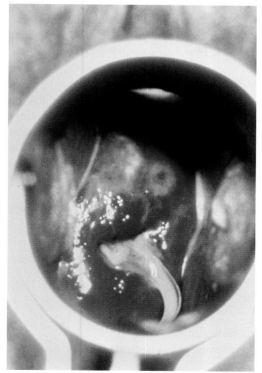

Figure 10-8. Viscous, opaque discharge emanating from the cervical os. (Photo contributed by Sue Rist, FNP, and reproduced with permission from Knoop KJ, Stack L, Storrow A, Thurman RJ. *The Atlas of Emergency Medicine*, 3rd ed., New York: McGraw-Hill; 2010.)

Which of the following is the next step in the management of this patient?

a. BHCG

b. Computed tomography (CT) of the abdomen

c. Chest radiography

d. Pelvic ultrasonography (US)

Answer a. BHCG

All women of childbearing age who are sexually active need a BHCG level. That is the first step to the workup. Pelvic US may be done after the BHCG result if it is positive. There is no need for chest radiography in this case. The same person who has enough unprotected sex to get an STD is the same person who has enough unprotected sex to get pregnant.

On the CCS, the initial order set should include BHCG, cervical swab and NAAT for Chlamydia and gonorrhea, and KOH wet prep.

Move the clock forward 1 hour.

Interval History: *The BHCG result is negative.*

What is the next step in the management of this patient?

a. Abdominal US

b. CT scan of the abdomen and pelvis

c. Await cervical cultures

d. Treat with azithromycin and ceftriaxone

e. Treat with ciprofloxacin and doxycycline

f. Treat with doxycycline and ceftriaxone

Answer f. Treat with doxycycline and ceftriaxone

Cervical motion tenderness that was noted on the physical examination means that the patient has PID. The patient should undergo immediate treatment. Waiting for the cultures to return is inappropriate; the patient needs treatment with antibiotics. The antibiotics of choice are doxycycline and ceftriaxone (Figure 10-9). Azithromycin can be successfully used for cervicitis or urethritis. It is not clear that azithromycin is acceptable for a deep-seated infection in the pelvis such as PID. No imaging is needed at this time because the infection can cause all of the patient's symptoms.

Quinolones are never to be considered acceptable for either gonorrhea or Chlamydia as first-line therapy.

Azithromycin is a macrolide.
• Activity against legionella, Chlamydia, campylobacter, and Enterobacteriaceae

Ceftriaxone is a third-generation cephalosporin.
• Activity against gram-positive and gram-negative bacteria

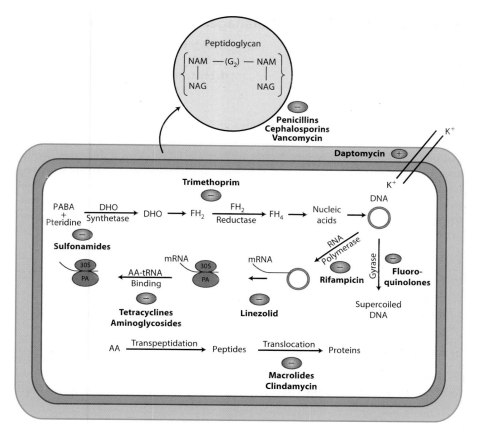

Figure 10-9. Mechanism of action of antibiotics. Penicillin, cephalosporins, and vancomycin work on the cell wall to prevent crosslinking. +, enhance; –, inhibit; aa, amino acid; DHO, dihydropteroate; FH2, dihydrofolate; FH4, tetrahydrofolate; G2, glucose; K+, potassium; PA, peptide donor-acceptor site. (Reproduced with permission from Tintinalli JE, Stapczynski J, Ma OJ, et al. *Tintinalli's Emergency Medicine: A Comprehensive Study Guide,* 7th ed. New York: McGraw-Hill; 2011.)

Move the clock forward 1 week.

Interval History: *The patient returns to the office 1 week later for worsening left lower quadrant abdominal pain. The patient states that she has also developed a fever and chills for the past 2 days.*

VS: *BP, 120/80 mm Hg; P, 95 beats/min; R, 16 breaths/min; T, 102.3°F*

PE:
- *Gen: Patient is writhing in pain*
- *Abd: Tenderness present in left lower quadrant, nondistended, bowel sounds normal*

What is the next step in the management of this patient?

a. CT of the abdomen
b. US of the pelvis

c. Magnetic resonance imaging (MRI) of the abdomen and pelvis
d. Hysterosalpingography

Answer b. US of the pelvis

US is the first-line imaging choice for patients with pelvic pain. US can detect abnormalities in the upper genital tract. CT of the abdomen would be indicated if there was concern for a gastrointestinal problem. The patient does not have any GI concerns at this time. The left lower quadrant pain is most likely associated with the PID for which the patient was being treated. MRI of the abdomen and pelvis is expensive and unnecessary when other modalities can visualize the genital tract. Hysterosalpingography would only show any abnormalities within the uterus and if the fallopian tubes are patent. It would not allow visualization of the ovaries.

> *Move the clock forward 2 hours.*
>
> **Interval History:** *Pelvic US shows a left-sided complex adnexal mass with surrounding inflammation. The mass itself is echogenic and contains fluid. It is consistent with an abscess larger than 10 cm in size.*
> *The patient continues to have pain in the left lower quadrant and remains febrile despite treatment with acetaminophen and ibuprofen.*
> *On the CCS, transfer the patient to the inpatient setting.*

What is the next step in the management of this patient?

a. Continue treatment with azithromycin and ceftriaxone
b. Change antibiotics to clindamycin and gentamicin

c. Change antibiotics to levofloxacin and metronidazole
d. Surgical drainage

Answer d. Surgical drainage

The patient has a tubo-ovarian abscess, a complication from PID. If the abscess ruptures, it is life-threatening emergency that can cause sepsis and death. Tubo-ovarian abscess should be treated with outpatient antibiotics if the following requirements are met:

- Less than 9 cm in size
- Patient is hemodynamically stable
- There is an adequate response to antibiotics
- Not postmenopausal

The following combinations are considered first-line antibiotic choices: cefoxitin and doxycycline or cefotetan and doxycycline. The combination of clindamycin and gentamicin is used when there is a life-threatening penicillin allergy such as anaphylaxis and even a cephalosporin should not be used. Notice that first-line therapy is a dual antibiotic regimen. Second-line therapy is levofloxacin and metronidazole. Because the first antibiotic regimen did not clear the infection, do not continue the same antibiotics.

Move the clock forward to the next day.

Interval History: *The patient had surgical drainage of the tubo-ovarian abscess. A total of 35 cc of pus was drained. The patient is now afebrile and no longer has any pain.*

CHAPTER 11

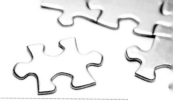

BREAST DISEASE

CASE 1: Benign Breast Mass

CC: "I feel a lump in my breast."

Setting: Outpatient office

VS: BP, 140/90 mm Hg; P, 90 beats/min; R, 16 breaths/min; T, 98.5°F

HPI: A 30-year-old woman presents for a breast mass she found in her right breast. The lump is painful, and she felt it 1 week before her menstruation. This has never happened before. Her grandmother had a history of breast cancer.

ROS:
- Denies fever, chills, and weight loss
- Denies chest pain, shortness of breath, abdominal pain, nausea, vomiting, diarrhea, and constipation

PE:
- Gen: awake, alert, oriented ×3, no acute distress
- Lungs: Clear to auscultation bilaterally
- Abd: Soft, nontender, nondistended, + bowel sounds
- Ext: No edema bilaterally
- Breasts: Symmetric, mobile masses bilaterally, nontender; largest mass on right breast (~3 cm by 3 cm)

What is the most likely diagnosis?

a. Fibrocystic changes
b. Fibroadenoma
c. Phylloides tumor

d. Mastitis
e. Intraductal papilloma

Answer a. Fibrocystic changes

Fibrocystic changes of the breast occur in up to 50% of women in the reproductive age. It is characterized by breast masses that change throughout the menstrual cycle. They often become painful and large just before menstruation. When menstruation occurs, the pain often resolves, and the masses regress. Fibroadenoma is a benign mass that is typically round, firm, mobile, and nontender. Phylloides tumor is a tumor that is not painful and often presents because of its rapid growth. These tumors cause some skin changes, a shiny stretched skin appearance, above the mass. Mastitis is an infection of the breast that causes a red, painful breast. It is basically cellulitis of the breast. Intraductal papilloma is a benign breast mass in the mammary ducts of the breast and often presents with bloody nipple discharge. This is a common type of breast mass in women ages 20 to 40 years.

What is the next step in management?

a. Biopsy of lesion

b. Breast ultrasonography (US)

c. Clinical breast examination alone

d. Mammogram

e. Biopsy

Answer b. Breast ultrasonography (US)

Clinical breast examination is not enough to establish a diagnosis. Mammography is less accurate in women younger than 40 years of age. Women younger than 40 years of age have denser breast tissue, making the mammogram harder to interpret. Biopsy of the lesion should be done, but imaging always comes first.

Breast US = Test of choice for women younger than 40 years old
Mammography = Test of choice for women older than 40 years old

---

Move the clock forward 1 week.

Interval History: *The patient states that she had the breast US done. She states that the masses seem smaller than previous, but the one on her right breast remains (Figure 11-1).*

Breast US report states that there are multiple fluid-filled cysts in each breast. The largest one (3 cm × 3 cm) is on the right side.

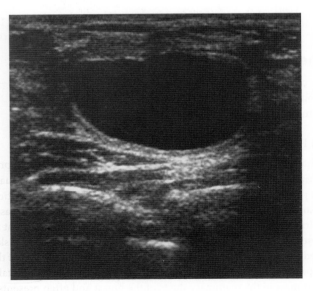

Figure 11-1. Ultrasonography of fibrocystic changes in breast. (Reproduced with permission from Chen MYM, et al. *Basic Radiology,* 2nd ed. McGraw-Hill, 2011.)

What is the next step in management?

a. Aspiration of the lesion

b. Excision of the mass

c. Repeat US in 6 months

d. Mammography

Answer a. Aspiration of the lesion

Although the diagnosis is still most likely fibrocystic changes of the breast, US shows a dominant mass or lesion. This dominant mass should undergo biopsy, or aspiration of the fluid. Excision of the mass is premature at this point; it is unclear what the mass is. Mammography is not used for evaluation of fluid-filled lesions. Mammography would not add anything to the US. Repeating the US in 6 months could have been done if there was no dominant mass or lesion. Biopsy will help distinguish between a mass (benign or malignant) and a cyst.

Fibroadenoma (Figure 11-2):
• Benign growth of breast
• Diagnosed on biopsy
• Not necessary to remove unless painful or rapidly growing

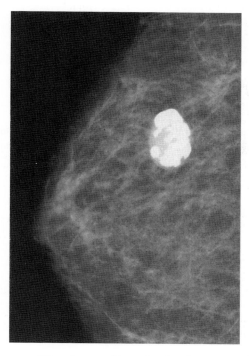

Figure 11-2. Mammogram of fibroadenoma. (Reproduced with permission from Chen MYM, et al. *Basic Radiology*, 2nd ed. McGraw-Hill, 2011.)

Move the clock forward 1 month.

Interval History: *The patient continues to have painful lumps in her breast during the premenstrual time of her cycle.*
Biopsy results show fibrosis of the dominant mass.

What is the treatment for fibrocystic disease of the breast?

a. Acetaminophen

b. Coffee

c. Oral contraceptive pills (OCPs)

d. Surgical intervention

e. Repeated aspirations of cysts

Answer c. Oral contraceptive pills (OCPs)

OCPs improve symptoms in up to 90% of patients. Caffeine should be avoided in fibrocystic disease of the breast. Nonsteroidal antiinflammatory drugs (NSAIDs) such as ibuprofen are the treatments of choice in adolescents. Tamoxifen and danazol also help. Surgical intervention or repeated aspirations of the cyst is not indicated in this benign disease.

Treatment of fibrocystic changes:
- Avoid caffeine
- Tamoxifen
- Danazol
- NSAIDs
- OCPs

Move the clock forward 6 months.

Interval History: *The patient states that after starting OCPs, the lumps slowly resolved. The patient no longer has painful and lumpy breasts before menstruation.*

CASE 2: Nipple Discharge

CC: " I have nipple discharge."

Setting: Outpatient office

VS: BP, 120/78 mm Hg; P, 85 beats/min; R, 15 breaths/min

HPI: A 25-year-old woman with no PMH, no PSH, and no allergies presents for unilateral nipple discharge. The patient states that it started about 3 weeks ago, appears whitish, and is unilateral. She does not think she felt any changes in her breast. She denies relation to her menstruation and uses condoms for contraception. She has never been pregnant and her last menstrual period (LMP) was 2 weeks ago.

ROS:
- Denies fever, chills, and weight loss
- Denies chest pain, shortness of breath, abdominal pain, nausea, vomiting, diarrhea, and constipation

PE:
- Gen: Awake, alert, oriented ×3, no acute distress
- CVS: S_1S_2+ RRR no m/r/g
- Lungs: Clear to auscultation bilaterally
- Abdomen: Soft, nontender, nondistended, + bowel sounds
- Ext: No edema bilaterally
- Breasts: Symmetric, no masses palpated, clear/whitish fluid expressed on manipulation of left breast.

What is the next step in the management of this patient?

a. Breast US

b. Thyroid-stimulating hormone (TSH) level

c. Prolactin level

d. Mammography

e. Refer to breast surgeon

Answer a. Breast US

The reasons for white discharge from the nipples are galactorrhea, lactation, and intraductal carcinomas. Endocrinologic causes usually cause bilateral nipple discharge. US is the test of choice. Mammography would be the first-line screening in patients older than 30 years old. Women younger than 30 years of age have very dense breast tissue, so US has better sensitivity and specificity. TSH and prolactin levels should be done if there is *bilateral* nipple discharge because bilateral nipple discharge is generally an endocrinologic etiology.

Unilateral discharge = Imaging
Bilateral discharge = Laboratory work (CMP, TSH, prolactin level, pregnancy test)

Interval History: *Breast US reveals a 4 cm × 4 cm mass in the left breast.*

What is the next step in the management of this patient?

a. Biopsy of the mass

b. Repeat US in 6 months

c. Repeat US in 1 year

d. Mammography in 6 months

e. Mammography in 1 year

Answer a. Biopsy of the mass

US-guided biopsy of a mass is always indicated if a mass is seen. Repeat imaging will prolong the time to diagnosis if it is cancer and is not indicated.

Interval History: *Biopsy shows intraductal papilloma, and the patient undergoes surgical intervention and treatment.*

CASE 3: Screening Examination

CC: *"I'm here for my routine physical exam."*

Setting: *Outpatient office*

VS: *BP, 120/80 mm Hg; P, 80 beats/min; R, 17 breaths/min; T, 98.7°F*

HPI: *A 50-year-old woman with no PMH presents for a routine physical examination. The patient states that she has been pregnant three times. She has two children who were born full term and delivered vaginally. She had one miscarriage. She has been with her husband for the past 23 years. The patient started her menstruation at 15 years old and is currently going through perimenopause. Her LMP was 3 months ago. The patient states that she last had a Pap smear 2 years ago. All of her Pap smears have been normal.*

ROS:
• *Denies any complaints*

PE:
• *Thyroid: Normal to palpation*
• *Breast: Symmetric, nontender, no lesions felt, no nipple inversion*
• *Cervix: Appears normal, no lesions seen*

Which of the following is the next best step in the management of this patient?

a. Vaginal culture

b. Nucleic acid amplification testing (NAAT) for Chlamydia

c. Potassium hydroxide (KOH) prep

d. Mammography

e. *BRCA* testing

Answer d. Mammography

At 50 years old, a woman should be having yearly mammography regardless of the clinical breast examination. Vaginal cultures and KOH are not indicated unless there is vaginal discharge; they are not routinely done. NAAT for Chlamydia is indicated as a screening test in women younger than the age of 25 years who have high-risk sexual practices. *BRCA* testing is done in women who have multiple family members with breast and ovarian cancer.

According to the U.S. Preventive Task Force (USPSTF), screening for breast cancer should be done starting at age 50 years and should stop at age 75 years. The decision to start mammograms earlier than age 50 years should be individualized. The USPSTF recommends against teaching women the self breast examination. USMLE will not get into the controversy about whether mammography should be routinely done between ages 40 to 50 years. Just as in this case, the answer will be clear. This patient needs a mammogram.

Interval History: *Mammogram returns with a Breast Imaging Reporting and Data System (BiRADS) 3.*

What is the next step in the management of this patient?

a. Repeat mammography now
b. Repeat mammography in 6 months
c. Repeat mammography yearly
d. US of breast
e. Biopsy of breast

Answer b. Repeat mammography in 6 months

The following is a chart of the BiRADS significance and when to follow up.

BIRADS Number	Significance	Follow-up
0	Incomplete visualization	Additional view needed with ultrasonography (US)
1	Negative	Routine yearly mammography
2	Benign findings	Routine yearly mammography
3	Probably benign findings	Repeat mammography in 6 months
4	Suspicious finding	US of breast and biopsy are needed
5	Highly suggestive of malignancy	US of breast and biopsy are needed
6	Biopsy-proven malignancy	Biopsy positive for cancer

Interval History: *The patient follows up for repeat mammography 6 months later. The mammogram report returns BiRADS 1 with yearly follow-up.*

CASE 4: Malignant Breast Mass

CC: *"I have a lump."*

Setting: *Outpatient office*

VS: *BP, 136/82; P, 73 beats/min; R, 18 breaths/min; T, 98.6°F*

HPI: *A 52-year-old woman with a past medical history of hypertension presents for a lump in her breast. The patient noticed that her left breast was becoming slightly deformed and appears swollen on one side. The patient states that she first realized it when she was getting dressed about a month ago. She thought that it would go away on its own, but it seems to be growing. She is very concerned.*

ROS:
• *Denies weight loss, pain in the breast, nipple discharge, and erythema of the breast*
• *Denies chest pain, shortness of breath, and abdominal pain*

PE:
• *Gen: Awake, alert, oriented ×3, no acute distress*
• *Breasts: Asymmetric. Left breast slightly larger than right, with mass on left upper outer quadrant of breast. Thickening of skin in the same area. Palpation significant for a 2 in × 3 in mass in the left upper outer quadrant, nontender, nonmobile. The right breast is unremarkable.*

Which of the following the next step in the management of this patient?

a. Wait 3 months and reevaluate the breast

b. Mammography

c. Mastectomy

d. Lumpectomy

e. US

Answer b. Mammography

Mammography is the best next step in the management of this patient. In reality, mammography, US, and biopsy would be ordered right away. However, for the test, mammography should be done first. US would be done first if the patient was younger than 40 years old. Invasive measures such as mastectomy and lumpectomy are never the first step. A patient with a breast lump should not be told to return in 3 months for reevaluation.

The upper outer quadrants are most likely to be the home of breast cancers (Figure 11-3).

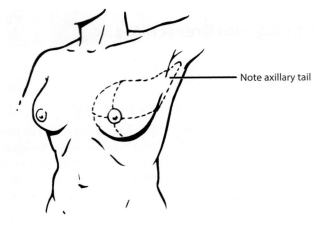

Note axillary tail

Figure 11-3. Breast quadrants. (Reproduced with permission from LeBlond RF, Brown D, DeGowin R. *DeGowin's Diagnostic Examination,* 9th ed. McGraw-Hill, 2009.)

Interval History: *Mammography results are BiRADS 4.*

Which of the following is the next best step in the management of this patient?

a. Core-needle biopsy

b. Bilateral mastectomy

c. Radical unilateral mastectomy

d. Computed tomography (CT) of the chest

Answer a. Core-needle biopsy

A biopsy of the suspected mass should be done before staging with CT of chest, or treatment with mastectomy. Biopsy is the next logical step in the sequence. Just because a mammogram suspects a malignant lesion does not mean that one is present. Biopsy must be done to confirm malignant properties. Mammography is done before core-needle biopsy because the biopsy itself will create abnormalities on the mammogram.

Core biopsy is more accurate than a needle biopsy and more deforming to the breast. Fine-needle biopsy is less sensitive but less complicated as well.

Interval History: *Biopsy returns with malignant cells. Surgical intervention is required. CT scan of the chest, abdomen, and pelvis are done. Tumor stage was found to be stage II. The patient will be referred to oncology and a breast surgeon.*

CASE 5: BRCA Gene

CC: *"I'm here for my routine physical examination."*

Setting: *Outpatient office*

HPI: *A 32-year-old generally healthy woman presents to the office for a routine pre-employment physical. She uses a vaginal ring for birth control. Her LMP was 2 weeks ago. She has been pregnant three times and has had two full-term births via normal spontaneous vaginal delivery. She had one spontaneous miscarriage at 10 weeks' gestation. She is only sexually active with her husband. She has a family history of breast cancer in her mother. Her mother had breast cancer at age 40 years and again at age 56 years. Her aunt also had breast cancer at an early age. Her last Pap smear, including human papillomavirus (HPV) was negative last year.*

VS: *BP, 120/80 mm Hg; P, 75 beats/min; R, 14 breaths/min; T, 98.4°F*

PE:
- *Gen: Awake, alert, oriented ×3*
- *CVS: $S_1 S_2$+ RRR no m/r/g*
- *Lungs: Clear to auscultation bilaterally*
- *Breast: No breast mass felt*

What should be done as a part of the evaluation?

a. Gonorrhea screening
b. Chlamydia screening
c. *BRCA* gene testing
d. Mammography
e. Pap smear

Answer c. *BRCA* gene testing

Gonorrhea and Chlamydia screening is only done routinely in women who are high risk or younger than 25 years of age. Pap smear is not necessary yearly in this age group, as long as all of her Pap smears have been normal and HPV testing was done. *BRCA* gene testing should be screened in all patients. This patient fulfills two of the risk factors, breast cancer in a family member younger than 45 years of age and multiple breast cancers in the same person (patient or relative).

Risk factors for *BRCA* gene:
1. Breast cancer at 45 years old or younger
2. Multiple breast cancers within the same person
3. Ovarian cancer at any age
4. Two relatives in the same side of the family with breast cancer (one younger than 50 years of age)

5. Three relatives in the same side of the family with breast cancer (any age)
6. Male breast cancer
7. Ashkenazi Jewish family with breast, ovarian, or pancreatic cancer in same side of family
8. Pancreatic cancer, ovarian cancer, or breast cancer in the same side of family
9. Triple negative breast cancer younger than the age of 60 years (no hormonal receptor status)
10. Known family member with *BRCA* gene

If two of these risk factors is positive, the patient should be screened for the *BRCA* gene.

Interval History: *The patient agreed to have the BRCA gene testing done. The test returns 6 weeks later. The result is positive.*

What is the next step in the management of this patient?

a. Mammography screening at 50 years old

b. Mammography now

c. Tamoxifen now

d. CA-125 screening at 40 years old

Answer b. Mammography now

Patients with a *BRCA* gene mutation are at a significantly increased risk of developing cancer. The reason for testing is to know if the patient is at increased risk, so that surveillance can be started earlier. It is recommended in patients with a positive *BRCA* gene that mammography begins at 25 years old. Screening mammography at age 50 years is done for the general population. Tamoxifen and CA-125 screening are still controversial in this population. Tamoxifen is used if the patient has two first-degree relatives such as a mother and a sister with breast cancer. Tamoxifen in that population can reduce the risk of breast cancer by 50%.

If the *BRCA* gene test result was negative, women are still at risk secondary to their familial risks.

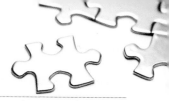

CHAPTER 12

CERVICAL ABNORMALITIES

CASE 1: Benign Cervical Growth

CC: *"I am here for my routine physical exam."*

Setting: *Outpatient office*

VS: *BP, 125/75 mm Hg; P, 75 beats/min; R, 16 breaths/min; T, 98.5°F*

HPI: *A 25-year-old woman presents for her routine gynecologic visit. She has been sexually active for the past year with one woman partner. She has never had a Pap smear. She denies ever having sexual relations with a man. The patient denies pain, abnormal vaginal bleeding, and pain during sexual relations. She has never been pregnant or had a sexually transmitted disease (STD).*

ROS: *Denies abdominal pain, nausea, vomiting, pelvic pain, vaginal bleeding, and vaginal discharge.*

The cervical examination is significant for which of the following, as shown below?

a. Nabothian gland cyst

b. Ectropion

c. Polyp

d. Bartholin gland cyst

Answer a. Nabothian gland cyst

A nabothian gland cyst is a benign growth on the outside of the cervix. There is no need to treat these cysts if they are asymptomatic.

Abnormality	Image	Treatment
Nabothian gland cyst: raised, symmetric, yellow lesion	(Reproduced with permission from Hoffman BL, Schorge J, Halvorson L, et al (eds). *Williams Gynecology*, 2nd ed. New York: McGraw-Hill; 2012.)	None if asymptomatic Symptomatic = removal If removed, scaring may lead to dyspareunia

(Continued)

Abnormality	Image	Treatment
Ectropion: visible columnar cells outside the internal os	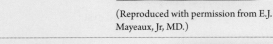 (Reproduced with permission from E.J. Mayeaux, Jr, MD.)	No treatment Common in adolescents, pregnant women, or women taking oral contraceptive pills
Polyp	(Reproduced with permission from E.J. Mayeaux, Jr, MD.)	Removal if >3 cm, bleeding, or appear atypical
Bartholin gland cyst	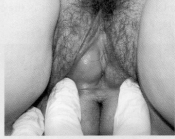 (Reproduced with permission from Hoffman BL, Schorge J, Halvorson L, et al (eds). *Williams Gynecology,* 2nd ed. New York: McGraw-Hill; 2012.)	I&D with Word catheter

What is the next step in the management of this patient?

a. Breast ultrasonography (US)   **c.** Pap smear
b. Gonorrhea screening

Answer c. Pap smear

Pap smear should be recommended starting at age 21 years regardless of sexual activity. Even if the patient has never had sex, a Pap smear should still be done. Breast US and gonorrhea screening are not routinely done. Chlamydia screening is done routinely until age 25 years.

Pap smear should be started at age 21 years regardless of sexual activity.

Sexual orientation does not matter in Pap smear guidelines. Human papillomavirus (HPV) may be transmitted during homosexual acts as well.

Pap smear is an evaluation of the cells that are scraped from the cervix.

Interval History: *Pap smear returned 4 weeks later negative for cervical cancer.*

CASE 2: Malignant Cervical Disease

CC: *"I have bleeding during sexual relations."*

Setting: *Outpatient office*

VS: *BP, 120/65 mm Hg; P, 82 beats/min; R, 15 breaths/min; T, 98.6°F*

HPI: *A 32-year-old woman presents for vaginal bleeding during intercourse. She has had more than 10 lifetime partners, both men and women. She has had a history of STD, such as chlamydia in her early 20s. The patient states that the vaginal bleeding is getting worse, and it is starting to occur at times other than after sex.*

ROS:
- *Denies weight loss, change in appetite, and fatigue*
- *Denies vaginal pain, tenderness, and dyspareunia*

PE:

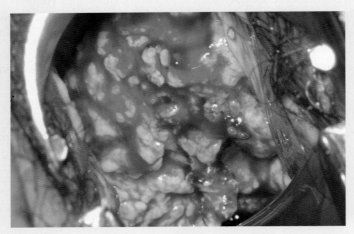

Figure 12-1. Cervical squamous cell carcinoma seen on the speculum examination. (Reproduced with permission from Daron Ferris, MD.)

What is the next step in the management of this patient?

a. Culture the bloody fluid

b. Total abdominal hysterectomy

c. Pap smear

d. Start chemotherapy

e. Computed tomography (CT) scan of the pelvis and abdomen

Answer c. Pap smear

When a red, friable, and bleeding cervix is encountered, it is likely that cervical carcinoma is the diagnosis. However, the diagnosis must be made with a Pap smear. The Pap smear will take some of the cells and observe their cellular qualities. Culture of the bloody fluid will not allow diagnosis of cancer but maybe of a bacterial infection as well. Treatment with both a total abdominal hysterectomy and chemotherapy is premature without a diagnosis of cervical carcinoma. CT scan of the abdomen and pelvis will be done when the Pap smear results return so that surgical intervention can be planned.

Which of the following is a risk factor for cervical cancer?

a. First intercourse at the age of 21 years
b. Immunocompromised state
c. One sexual partner
d. High socioeconomic status
e. First baby at age 21 years

Answer b. Immunocompromised state

Immunocompromised states such as HIV/AIDS are a risk for cervical cancer. Cervical cancer is caused by the HPV virus. When the body is unable to clear the virus, as in an immunocompromised state, the patient is more likely to be affected.

Risk factors for cervical cancer:
• Early onset of sexual activity (<21 years old)
• Multiple sexual partners
• High-risk partner (has HPV)
• Immunocompromised
• History of sexually transmitted infection (STI)
• History of vulvar lesions or warts (related to HPV)
• Early age of first birth (<21)
• Multiparity (>three children)
• Low socioeconomic status

Which of the following describes the virus that most commonly causes cervical cancer?

a. Double-stranded RNA virus
b. Nonenveloped DNA virus
c. Enveloped DNA virus
d. Positive-sense single-stranded RNA virus

Answer b. Nonenveloped DNA virus

HPV is a nonenveloped DNA virus. Double-stranded RNA virus example is rotavirus. Poliovirus, rubella virus, yellow fever virus, and rhinovirus are all positive-sense single-stranded RNA viruses. Poxviruses are enveloped DNA viruses.

HPV strands known to cause cancer:
• 16, 18, 31, 33, 35, 39, 45, 51, 52, 56, 58, 59, 68, 69, and 82

Move the clock forward 3 weeks.

Interval History: *The Pap smear results indicate high-grade squamous intraepithelial lesion (HSIL).*

What is the next step in the management of this patient?

a. Total abdominal hysterectomy

b. Colposcopy

c. Loop electrosurgical excision (LEEP)

d. Observe and repeat screening in 6 months

Answer b. Colposcopy

HSIL is a classification that encompasses anything from CIN2 through carcinoma in situ. The patient may have severe dysplasia or carcinoma. The only way to distinguish between these two is by colposcopy. Observation and repeat screening in 6 months is not recommended because HSIL may be carcinoma and need treatment. LEEP and total abdominal hysterectomy are treatment options depending on the diagnosis of cancer and the extent of the lesions.

> Colposcopy is a diagnostic test in which the tissue of the vagina, vulva, and cervix are magnified and lesions are better seen (Figure 12-2). Biopsies may also be taken at this time.

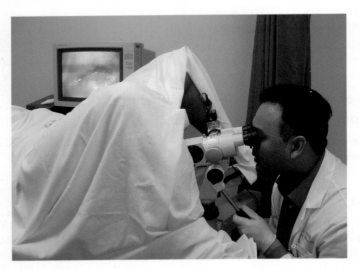

Figure 12-2. Colposcopy. (Reproduced with permission from E.J. Mayeaux, Jr, MD.)

Interval History: *Colposcopy results return with CIN1.*

What is the next best step in the management of this patient?

a. Repeat colposcopy in 6 months

b. HPV testing in 1 year

c. Repeat Pap smear and HPV testing in 12 months

d. Return to normal screening as per age guidelines

Answer c. Repeat Pap smear and HPV testing in 12 months

Biopsy is more accurate than a Pap smear; therefore, when the colposcopy biopsy results return with CIN1, there are a couple choices in management. One option is to repeat the HPV and Pap smear at 12 and 24 months. The other choice is to do an excisional diagnostic procedure, such as LEEP or cone biopsy.

LEEP = Loop electrosurgical excision (Figure 12-3)

Interval History: *Repeat Pap smear done 1 year later shows normal cytology but is positive for HPV.*

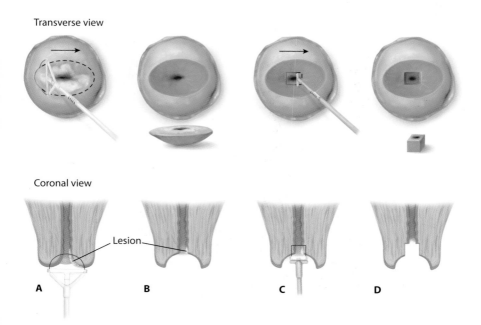

Transverse view

Coronal view

Lesion

A   B   C   D

Figure 12-3. Steps to loop electrosurgical excision procedure. (Reproduced with permission from Hoffman BL, Schorge J, Halvorson L, et al (eds). *Williams Gynecology,* 2nd ed. New York: McGraw-Hill; 2012.)

What is the next step in the management of this patient?

a. Repeat Pap smear in 6 months

b. Repeat Pap smear in 1 year

c. Colposcopy

d. LEEP

Answer c. Colposcopy

When a repeat Pap smear is done in 1 year, if HPV is positive or there is a cytologic abnormality (except HSIL), then a colposcopy should be performed. If HSIL was present on the repeat Pap smear, a LEEP or other excisional diagnostic study should be performed. Repeating the Pap smear in 6 months would not be an option. If the HPV result was negative and cytology result was negative on this Pap smear, another repeat Pap smear should be done in 1 year.

Interval History: *Colposcopy was done, and the results were normal. The patient will have a repeat Pap smear in 12 months.*

CASE 3: Abnormal Pap Smear Findings

Setting: *Outpatient office*

CC: *"I am here for my routine visit."*

VS: *BP, 120/80 mm Hg; P, 83 beats/min; R, 15 breaths/min; T, 98.3°F*

HPI: *A 28-year-old woman presents to the office for her routine Pap smear. She has had eight lifetime partners but has recently gotten married. For the past 5 years, she has only been sexually active with her husband. All of her previous Pap smear results have been normal. She denies any history of STIs. She has never been pregnant, although she would like to become pregnant soon. She denies any vaginal discharge, abnormal vaginal bleeding, or dyspareunia.*

ROS: *Entire ROS is negative*

PE: *Pelvic examination was done. Pap smear completed. No cervical discharge, no cervical lesions present.*

Bimanual Exam: *No cervical motion tenderness, no adnexal enlargement or tenderness, no uterine enlargement*

What is the next step in the management of this patient?

a. Discuss birth control options

b. Start folic acid supplementation

c. Gonorrhea and Chlamydia screening

Answer b. Start folic acid supplementation

The patient stated that she would like to become pregnant soon. All women who are interested in becoming pregnant should have folic acid supplementation. Women can start to take prenatal vitamins or folic acid alone. The body should have enough folic acid before the patient realizes that she is pregnant in order to prevent neural tube defects. Birth control options should be discussed with patients who are not considering getting pregnant. Chlamydia screening is done yearly until age 25 years. After age 25 years, it is done in high-risk groups. This patient would not qualify as high risk.

Interval History: *The patient's Pap smear results indicate ASC-US (atypical squamous cells of undetermined significance).*

Which of the following is the next step in the management of this patient?

a. Repeat Pap smear in 6 months

b. Repeat Pap smear in 2 years

c. HPV testing now

d. Colposcopy

Answer c. HPV testing now

Often when a patient's Pap smear indicate ASC-US, a reflex HPV test is done. However, if it was not, HPV testing is the preferred next step. If HPV testing is not done, a repeat Pap in 1 year is also acceptable. Colposcopy and routine screening would be considered if the HPV status was known.

Interval History: *HPV testing was done and results are negative.*

Which of the following is the next step in the management of this patient?

a. Repeat Pap in 1 year

b. Repeat Pap and HPV in 1 year

c. Repeat Pap and HPV in 3 years

d. Colposcopy

Answer c. Repeat Pap and HPV in 3 years

Even though the Pap smear returned with some atypical cells, the HPV (the most common cause for cervical cancer) result is negative. If the HPV result is negative, the patient can resume normal screening with HPV co-testing. Screening at ages 25 years and older is done every 3 years. Pap smear and HPV testing are no longer indicated in a year. Pap smear with HPV testing is done every 5 years when the patient turns 30 years.

If HPV testing was not done, a Pap smear could have been repeated in 1 year, but with a negative HPV screening, a Pap in 1 year is no longer needed. If the HPV result returned positive in a 25-year-old patients, a colposcopy would have been recommended. A patient between the ages of 21 and 24 years is managed slightly differently. If the patient had a Pap smear that returned with ASC-US, either repeat Pap smear in 12 months or HPV could be done. If the HPV result was positive, a repeat Pap smear, not a colposcopy, would be done in 12 months. The guidelines for younger patients are more conservative because it is often found that the patients will clear the HPV infection on their own.

Age of the patient is imperative in ASC-US management:
- 21 to 24 years = Repeat Pap smear in 12 months (even if HPV positive)
- 25 years+ = HPV testing (preferred) or repeat Pap smear in 12 months
  - If positive HPV = Colposcopy
  - If negative HPV = Repeat Pap smear and HPV in 3 years

CASE 4: Screening Examination and Vaccination

Setting: *Outpatient office*

CC: *"I'm here for my routine visit."*

VS: *BP, 116/70 mm Hg; P, 82 beats/min; R, 15 breaths/min; T, 98.7°F*

HPI: *A 20-year-old woman with no PMH presents for her annual physical examination. She has been sexually active for the past 3 years with five lifetime partners. She has never been to an ob/gyn. She has had all of her vaccinations: MMR (mumps, measles, and rubella), varicella, hepatitis A and B, DTaP (diphtheria, tetanus, and pertussis).*

ROS: *Denies vaginal discharge, vaginal itching, and sexual dysfunction*

PE: *Pelvic examination findings are within normal limits*

Which of the following should be recommended?

a. Pap smear

b. HPV vaccination

c. Gonorrhea screening

Answer b. HPV vaccination

HPV vaccination is recommended to girls and women starting at age 11 years. The vaccine has been found to be more effective before women become infected with HPV, but it is recommended until the age of 26 years regardless of sexual activity. It is given in a three-shot series. Pap smear is not recommended until age 21 years regardless of the patient's sexual activity. Gonorrhea is not screened for alone in patients. Chlamydia screening is recommended to patients until age 25 years.

Pap Smear recommendations
- Start at age 21 years regardless of sexual activity
- Pap smear alone every 3 years
           or
- Pap smear with HPV every 5 years (if >30 years old)
- Stop screening if normal Pap smear results at age 65 years
- No Pap smear in women who have had a total hysterectomy (no cervix) for noncancerous reasons

The patient opts to have the HPV vaccination, and it is administered at this time.

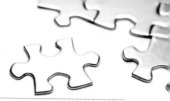

OVARIAN DISEASE

CASE 1: Ovarian Torsion

CC: *"I have abdominal pain."*

Setting: *Emergency department*

VS: *BP, 140/90 mm Hg; P, 90 beats/min; R, 15 breaths/min; T, 98.4°F*

HPI: *A 32-year-old woman presents to the emergency department for left lower quadrant abdominal pain for the past 2 days. The patient states the pain is 8 of 10 on the pain scale, non-radiating, and started off intermittent. The pain is now constant. She denies vomiting, diarrhea, and constipation but has nausea intermittently. Her last menstrual period was around 3 or 4 weeks ago. She has one sexual partner, and they have been trying to get pregnant.*

ROS: *Negative except for above.*

PE:
• *Abd: Soft, tender in the left lower quadrant on palpation, + bowel sounds*

Which of the following is the next step in the management of this patient?

a. Beta-human chorionic gonadotropin (BHCG)

b. Computed tomography (CT) scan of the abdomen and pelvis

c. Complete blood count (CBC)

d. Transvaginal ultrasonography (US)

Answer a. Beta-human chorionic gonadotropin (BHCG)

BHCG is the first step in any woman of childbearing age. In real life, its possible to order the CBC, BHCG, and imaging at the same time. BHCG will help to rule out ectopic pregnancy. CBC may be helpful in distinguishing if there is an infectious component to the process but does not rule any diagnosis in or out. Imaging may be done, but it must first be established if the patient is pregnant.

Differential diagnosis:
• Ectopic pregnancy
• Tubo-ovarian abscess
• Ovarian cyst
• Appendicitis if on right side

The BHCG test results are negative.

Which of the following is the test of choice for this patient?

a. CT of the abdomen and pelvis
b. Magnetic resonance imaging (MRI) of the abdomen and pelvis
c. Transabdominal US

Answer c. Transabdominal US

A differential diagnosis should be established for each patient who presents to the physician. In this particular case, one would think there is something in the pelvis because the patient does not have gastrointestinal symptoms. One should be suspicious for pelvic causes of left lower quadrant pain, such as ovarian cyst, ovarian torsion, or ovarian mass. Nausea is common with all of these etiologies. MRI of the abdomen and pelvis is never the first-line imaging. CT of the abdomen and pelvis may be done and often picks up on ovarian causes when the test is done for other reasons. However, the test of choice for ovarian etiology is US.

Test of choice for ovarian torsion: US

US results show an enlarged and edematous left ovary compared with the right. There is also a 5-cm cystic mass on the left ovary. Doppler of the left ovary shows decreased blood flow.

Which of the following is the next step in the management of this patient?

a. Serial US of the ovary
b. Salpingo-oophorectomy

c. Laparotomy with detorsion
d. Exploratory laparotomy

Answer c. Laparotomy with detorsion

This patient is a young woman in her reproductive years who wants to get pregnant. The mass on the ovary is a cyst and is large enough to cause the torsion of the ovary. Conservative management with detorsion should be attempted first. Only if that is not possible should the ovary and fallopian tube be removed in a procedure called a salpingo-oophorectomy.

An exploratory laparotomy is not needed because we know the etiology of the pain. Serial US of the ovaries is only necessary when ovarian masses are found in fetuses and infants. Ovarian torsion is an emergency; serial US is not warranted.

Risk factors for torsion:
- Ovarian mass >5 cm in size
- Reproductive age
- Pregnancy
- Ovulation induction
- Prior torsion

Treatment:
- Must detorse (untwist) the ovary immediately
- In patients of reproductive age, try to save ovary, including by cystectomy
- In postmenopausal age, may remove ovary and fallopian tube (salpingo-oophorectomy)

The patient had a detorsion and cystectomy, and her ovary was preserved.

CASE 2: Benign Ovarian Disease

CC: *"I have abdominal pain."*

Setting: *Outpatient office*

VS: *BP, 122/84 mm Hg; P, 90; R, 13 breaths/min; T, 98.7°F*

HPI: *A 34-year-old woman with no PMH presents to the office for intermittent left lower quadrant pain, nonradiating for the past 24 hours. She had her menstruation 1.5 weeks ago. She has no nausea, vomiting, diarrhea, or constipation. She denies dysuria, urinary urgency, and urinary frequency.*

ROS:
• *Denies fever, chills*
• *AS per HPI*

PE:
• *Abd: soft, nondistended, left lower quadrant tenderness is present on superficial and deep palpation. The pain radiates toward the midline.*

Which of the following is the next step in the management of this patient?

a. BHCG
b. Pelvic US
c. Abdominal CT

d. CBC
e. Morphine administration

Answer a. BHCG

The first test on any woman of childbearing age with abdominal pain is a pregnancy test. If this is one of the options, it is the correct answer.

Interval History: *The patient is still complaining of pelvic pain. The BHCG test result is negative.*

Which of the following is the next step in the management of this patient?

a. Abdominal CT
b. Abdominal US

c. Pelvic US
d. Pelvic MRI

Answer c. Pelvic US

Pelvic US is the imaging modality of choice in the evaluation of the pelvic mass or pain in women. Abdominal CT and US will not evaluate the pelvic structures as needed in the patient. Pelvic MRI may be needed, but US is always done first.

Move the clock forward 1 week.

Interval History: *US results are significant for a 4-cm simple cyst; the patient no longer has any pain.*

Which of the following is the next step in the management of this patient?

a. Repeat US in 8 weeks

b. Refer to ob/gyn

c. Pelvic MRI

d. CA-125

Answer a. Repeat US in 8 weeks

A simple cyst is one that is filled with fluid and has no solid components. Simple cysts are often follicular cysts. Follicular cysts are the most common types of cyst and may range in size from 3 to 8 cm. They are the result of a failure of the follicle to rupture in ovulation. These cysts often are asymptomatic until they become large. Large cysts may cause torsion of the ovary, which will in turn cause pain. These type of cysts are monitored by repeat US in 2 months. There should be spontaneous resolution within that time period.

Move the clock forward 2 months.

Repeat US was done, and another cyst was found on the other ovary.

Which of the following is the next step in the management of this patient?

a. CA-125

b. Oral contraceptive pills (OCPs)

c. Surgical removal

Answer b. Oral contraceptive pills (OCPs)

OCPs stop ovulation. If ovulation stops, then there is no follicle. If there is no follicle, then there can be no follicular cyst.

CA-125 is a tumor marker that is expressed in ovarian cancer. This is not indicated at this time because the original cyst has resolved, but a new cyst has formed. A CA-125 would be indicated if the original cyst had persisted or had the characteristics of a malignant tumor. Tumor markers such as CA-125 are not to determine a diagnosis. They are to allow follow-up in response to treatment.

Simple cysts most often do not need surgical removal. Aspiration was done in the past, but the cysts often recurred. As long as the follicular cyst is asymptomatic, no surgical intervention is needed.

Histology of follicular cyst:
• Inner layer of granulosa cells   • Outer layer of theca cells

Types of cysts:
• Follicular cysts (Figure 13-1)
• Corpus luteum cysts
• Theca lutein cysts
• Endometriomas (Figure 13-2)

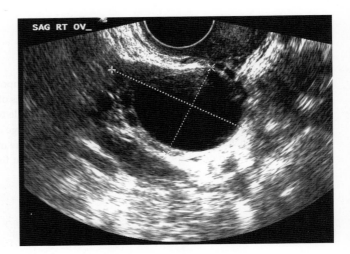

Figure 13-1. Follicular cyst on ultrasonography. (Reproduced with permission from Dr. Elysia Moschos.)

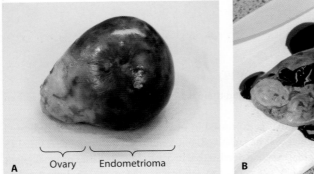

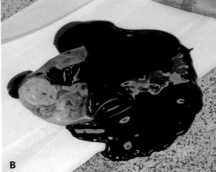

Figure 13-2. Endometrioma after surgical removal. (Reproduced with permission from Dr. Roxanne Pero.)

Interval History: *The patient was placed on OCPs and has not had anymore pelvic pain.*

CASE 3: Malignant Ovarian Disease

CC: " I have lower abdominal fullness."

Setting: Outpatient office

VS: BP, 110/70 mm Hg; P, 97; R, 18; T, 98.6°F

HPI: A 45-year-old woman with no PMH presents to the office for an increase in abdominal fullness and bloating, worsening over the past 3 or 4 months. The patient states that she feels nauseous all the time, although has not had any vomiting. She states because of the constant nausea, she has not been eating as much. She has had a 10-lb weight loss in the last 4 months.

ROS:
- Denies fever, chills
- Weight loss has occurred (10 lb in 4 months)
- Denies chest pain, shortness of breath, and abdominal pain
- Nausea is present with no vomiting
- No diarrhea or constipation

PE:
- Gen: Awake, alert, oriented ×3
- Abd: Soft, nontender, distended bowel sounds are present, shifting dullness to percussion is present
- Pelvic: Cervix normal, no cervical motion tenderness, right adnexal enlargement is present

Which of the following is the next step in the management of this patient?

a. Abdominal US

b. BHCG

c. Hepatitis panel

d. Pelvic US

e. CA-125

Answer: b. BHCG

Always do a BHCG in women of childbearing age first when presenting with abdominal symptoms. It is always the first step.

Patients with ovarian cancer often present late in the course with abdominal distention, adnexal masses, and vague constitutional symptoms. However, tubo-ovarian abscess and ectopic pregnancy are also in the differential diagnosis. If the patient was young, germ cell tumors should be considered.

Ovarian cancers often present in the late stages with abdominal pain, abdominal distention, bloating, and early satiety. The reason for the late presentation is the early symptoms are very nonspecific. Patients often do not present for evaluation during these vague symptoms. Ovarian cancers tend to spread via seeding onto the omentum. This metastasis is what causes the late symptoms.

Types of germ cell tumors:

Type of Germ Cell Tumor	Histology
Dysgerminoma	Large, round cells with central nuclei
Immature teratoma	Cells from three germ layers
Endodermal sinus tumors	Schiller-Duval bodies (single papilla lined with tumor cells and central blood vessel)
Embryonal carcinoma	Solid sheets of polygonal cells with eosinophilic cytoplasm
Choriocarcinoma	Cytotrophoblasts and syncytiotrophoblasts
Gonadoblastoma	Germ cells and sex cord cells surrounded by stroma
Mixed germ tumors	Two or more germ cell layers

Types of epithelial ovarian tumors:

Type of Tumor	Prevalence Among Epithelial Tumors	Histology
Serous cystadenoma	75%	Cystic structures with papilla that may extend into the cyst. Also have psammoma bodies
Mucinous cystadenoma	10%	Endocervical epithelium with hyperchromatic (darkened) nuclei
Endometrioid	10% 30% are bilateral	Glandular architecture
Clear cell	<1%	"Clear cells" (meaning no content)
Undifferentiated	<10%	No clear way to make a distinction

Move the clock forward 1 day.

The following laboratory examinations returned:
- *BHCG: Negative*
- *CBC: White blood cell (WBC) count, 5.3 × 10³/μL*
- *Hemoglobin: 10.3 g/dL*
- *Hematocrit: 31%*
- *Platelet count: 250 × 10³/μL*
- *CA-125: Elevated*

Which of the following is the next step in the management of this patient?

a. Refer to surgery for total abdominal hysterectomy

b. Pelvic US

c. Pelvic MRI

d. Ovarian biopsy

Answer b. Pelvic US

Even though the CA-125 level is elevated, it does not mean this is ovarian cancer. It is more likely, but just based on a CA-125 level, you would not do a total abdominal hysterectomy. The patient must first be evaluated for ovarian cancer. This is done with imaging first. You should not remove something without first confirming the etiology. Pelvic US is the imaging of choice because it has the least amount of radiation and is the least expensive. Pelvic MRI is never the initial choice for imaging. Ectopic pregnancy and tubo-ovarian abscess have been ruled out because the BHCG and WBC count are normal.

CA-125 levels are increase in:
- Pancreatic cancer
- Colon cancer
- Fallopian tube cancer

- Endometriosis
- Pelvic inflammatory disease

CA-125 is a mucin glycoprotein

Move the clock forward 1 week.

The pelvic US results show a right-sided complex mass with septations and solid components. Ascites is seen within the abdomen.

Which of the following is a risk factor for ovarian cancer?

a. Breastfeeding

b. OCP use

c. Age younger than 40 years

d. Infertility

Answer d. Infertility

The strongest risk factor for ovarian cancer is a family history. The *BRCA* gene is found to increase the lifetime risk of both ovarian cancers and breast cancers. Other risk factors include age, early menarche (first menstruation), late menopause, infertility, and nulligravidity (no children). Protective factors include OCP use and breastfeeding. The theory for the development of ovarian cancer is based on how often an egg is released. The more the egg is released and the epithelium needs to repair itself, the more likely it is to get a mutation.

Risk factors for ovarian cancer:
• Age (older than 40 years)
• Early menarche (first menstruation before 12 years old)
• Late menopause (after age 50 years)
• Whites have highest risk as an ethnicity
• Infertility
• Endometriosis
• Nulligravida (no children)
• Family history

Protective factors
• OCP use
• Breastfeeding

General population has a lifetime risk of 1.7%.
BRCA-positive patients have lifetime risk of 45%.

Move the clock forward 1 week.

Pelvic CT and MRI are done, showing widespread disease with metastasis. Surgical consultation is obtained, and surgical intervention is planned.

However, the patient comes to the office with severe abdominal pain, nausea, and vomiting. The patient has not had a bowel movement in 4 days.

VS: *BP, 145/80 mm Hg; P, 110 beats/min; R, 18 breaths/min; T, 100.5°F*

PE:
• *Gen: The patient is writhing in pain.*
• *CVS: S_1S_2 +, tachycardia*
• *Abdominal pain: Rigid, no BS present*

Which of the following is the next step in the management of this patient?

a. CBC

b. CMP

c. Abdominal CT scan

d. Chest radiography

Answer d. Chest radiography

On the CCS, the patient should be transferred to the emergency department. This patient is likely experiencing a complication to ovarian cancer, which includes abdominal obstruction and perforation. Chest radiography should be done along with the abdominal radiography to see if there is free air under the diaphragm. Abdominal CT may be done after the radiography if the radiography does not reveal free air. CBC and CMP should be drawn but will not give you a clear diagnosis.

Move the clock forward 10 minutes.

Chest radiography shows free air under the diaphragm.

VS: *BP, 100/80 mm Hg; P, 120 beats/min; R, 20 breath/min; T, 102.5°F*

Which of the following is the next step in the management of this patient?

a. Administer normal saline.

b. Administer metronidazole.

c. Await surgical consult.

Answer a. Administer normal saline.

This patient is in septic shock. To keep the circulatory system working, perfusion pressure should be addressed first. Administering normal saline will increase the blood pressure and hopefully slow down the heart rate. Antibiotics should be administered during surgery. Surgery is necessary to repair the perforation.

Move the clock forward 1 hour.

The patient is in surgery to repair the perforation.

CASE 4: Polycystic Ovarian Syndrome

CC: *"I have a lot of hair on my face."*

Setting: *Office*

VS: *BP, 130/80 mm Hg; P, 85 beats/min; R, 15 breaths/min; T, 98.7°F*

HPI: *A 24-year-old woman presents to the office for facial hair. The patient states that she has noticed facial hair starting to appear for the past month. She states that she has also been having an increase in her acne. The patient denies chest pain, shortness of breath, and abdominal pain. Menstruation has been irregular, and she has not had one in almost 6 months.*

ROS: *Denies chest pain, shortness of breath, abdominal pain, nausea, vomiting, diarrhea, and constipation*

PE:
- *Face: Moderate acne, facial hair around lip, sideburns, cheeks*
- *CVS: Normal*
- *Lungs: Normal*
- *Abd: Normal*
- *Ext: No edema*

Initial Orders:
- *Luteinizing hormone (LH) level*
- *Follicle-stimulating hormone (FSH) level*
- *DHEA (dehydroepiandrosterone) level*
- *Glucose and HgA1c level*

The patient returns in a week to discuss the results of the tests.
- *LH: Elevated*
- *FSH: Normal*
- *DHEA: Elevated*
- *Glucose: 112 mg/dL*
- *HgA1c: 6.2%*

Which of the following is the next step in the management of this patient?

a. Start the patient on metformin

b. Transvaginal US

c. Start OCPs

d. Start clomiphene

Answer c. Start OCPs

The diagnosis of polycystic ovarian syndrome (PCOS) is not actually based only on the visualization of the cystic ovaries. Two of the following three symptoms must be present: oligomenorrhea (or amenorrhea), hyperandrogenism, and polycystic ovaries on US. This patient has the secondary amenorrhea and the hyperandrogenism. Hirsutism is found in about 50% of PCOS patients, and 30% to 50% are obese. The patient was concerned with hirsutism, so the treatment would be OCPs. OCPs are the first-line treatment for women who do not desire children.

Polycystic ovaries on US = "String of pearls"

Histologically appear as fluid-filled follicles beneath a fibrous cortex

The patient was placed on OCPs. Over the next 6 months she continues to have hirsutism.

Which of the following is the next step in the management of this patient?

a. Double the dose of oral contraceptive.
b. Add spironolactone.
c. Start clomiphene.
d. Start flutamide.
e. Start diet and exercise program.

Answer b. Add spironolactone.

Doubling the dose of OCPs is never indicated. Clomiphene helps with infertility, not hirsutism. Spironolactone is given as a second-line treatment to help augment the OCPs. Flutamide is not second-line treatment secondary to hepatotoxicity.

Weight loss is indicated in the PCOS population to help decrease the metabolic risks; however, it has not been proven to have cosmetic effects. It should be given in women with insulin resistance.

Metformin is routinely used in PCOS.
First-line treatments include OCPs (for those who do not want children) and weight loss and clomiphene (for those wishing to have children).

The patient returns the following month with decrease acne and less abnormal facial hair.

INDEX

Page numbers followed by *f* or *t* indicate figures or tables, respectively.